THE BEST OF
TOTAL HEALTH

Edited by
ROBERT L. SMITH
Publisher of TOTAL HEALTH Magazine

A Division of GL Publications
Ventura, CA U.S.A.

Other good reading
> *How to Be Fit and Free* by Rick Kasper
> *Alcoholism* by Claire Costales with Jo Berry
> *Drug Abuse* by Loyd V. Allen, Jr.

The foreign language publishing of all Regal books is under the direction of Gospel Literature International (Glint). GLINT provides financial and technical help for the adaptation, translation and publishing of books for millions of people worldwide.

For information regarding translation, contact: GLINT, P.O. Box 6688, Ventura, California 93006.

Scripture quotations in this publication are from the *New American Standard Bible.* © The Lockman Foundation 1960, 1962, 1963, 1971, 1972, 1973, 1975. Used by permission. Other versions quoted are: the Authorized King James Version.
The Living Bible, Copyright © 1971 by Tyndale House Publishers, Wheaton, Illinois. Used by permission.

Articles in this publication are reprinted from *Total Health* magazine, Robert L. Smith, Editor-Publisher; used by permission.

Published by Regal Books
A Division of GL Publications
Ventura, California 93006
Printed in U.S.A.

Library of Congress Catalog Card No. 81-52940
ISBN 0-8307-0803-0

CONTENTS

INTRODUCTION

I am really delighted that you chose this book. It will definitely help you along the road to life's most important asset—good health!

There's a great day dawning. It's a holistic revolution and it really got started during the rebellion of the sixties when young people went back to the soil to raise their own fruits and vegetables and to bake their own whole-grain breads.

Now everybody's into natural food, jogging, body-building, positive thinking, prayer and meditation. We are discovering slowly the real purpose and meaning of life, accepting ourselves and loving others. This is the concept of *wholeness*.

And this is happening just in time. With hospital costs projected at $2,000 a day in just 15 years we need to begin a new self-help, preventive health program. This program should include educating the populace in diet, nutrition, fitness and in mental and spiritual health. This education should encompass home, family, school, church, state and federal government.

Everything we need for good health has been on this planet since creation. In the Old Testament God said, "Behold, I have given you every plant yielding seed that is on the surface of all the earth, and every tree which has fruit yielding seed; it shall be food for you" (Gen. 1:29). Now all we have to do is learn to raise and serve these simple foods and avoid the salt-and-sugar-filled, artificially-processed foods. Your body is bound to respond in a positive way to good nutrition combined with an exercise program.

I hope the concept of total health and wellness may become a way of life for you. After all, it's not the quantity of life that counts, it's the *quality*.

My 94-year-old mother has asked me many times, "I wonder how I will die? Will I have a stroke?" My reply, "Mom, you'll just go to sleep and not wake up. In other words, *you'll die well*!"

The chapters selected here are how-to guides to help you improve your health. They are from past issues of *Total Health* magazine, each selected for its practical value.

My hope is that you glean much information from this book, authored by some of this country's talented doctors, nutritionists, pastors and psychologists. If you would like more information about health, write: *Total Health* Magazine, 1800 N. Highland Avenue, Suite 720, Los Angeles, California, 90028.

Robert L. Smith
Editor-Publisher
Total Health Magazine

1

THE LOCKED HOOD

By Dr. Eppie Hartsuiker

Collectors of automobiles refer to the years 1925 to 1942 as the classic years— a period when the luxurious, fast motorcars reached their zenith. The first name in this field was Rolls-Royce—a name synonymous with wealth and prestige. These Rolls-Royce machines were so expensive that it was reportedly said that if you asked its price you couldn't afford one. This British car-manufacturing company, founded in 1904, designed its chassis primarily for limousine and large bodies which were not only noted for their speed (90 to 130 miles or 140 to 210 kilometers per hour) but for their luxurious comfort. They were limited in luxury only by the purse or checkbook of the buyer. The great custom coach builders of England furnished the bodies for Rolls-Royce motorcars. These artisans were prepared to satisfy any request, whether for upholstery in matched ostrich hide or for a dashboard in rosewood.

But most unique of the Rolls-Royce manufacturing practices was the locking of the bonnet, better known to Americans as the hood of the car. And the key remained in the custody of the company. In no other way could the

Rolls-Royce company be more assured that only their qualified technicians would have access to their superb motor. One could say that the purchaser might own the car, but the motor belonged to the Rolls-Royce company. Whenever the car malfunctioned (perish the thought) or was in need of repair, it was driven or hauled into their repair shop, the hood unlocked by their technicians and repaired. However, this unique and sensible method of thwarting the mishandling of their motor is no longer in vogue. In fact, the Rolls-Royce is no longer the envied symbol of the titled and the exclusive only.

However, whether the Rolls-Royce people realized it or not they were only following a unique system of maintenance and supervision of divine wisdom.

We are entering into an era of self-care—that is, being more responsible for our health. This is paradoxical in that we have more technological skill and medical science know-how than any other period of history, with perhaps the exception of the ancients. This awareness of taking an active part in the care of one's health may be due to the rising cost of health care, or the realization that physicians are not miracle men and women, or the belief that we are owned of God and as good stewards are responsible for the proper care of our bodies.

The projected figures for future health care are mind-boggling. In fact they are downright scary. Can you imagine paying over $2,000 a day for a hospital bed? Yet this is the projected cost by the end of this century! And in spite of the wonders of organ transplants, test-tube babies, smallpox eradication, the decline of infectious diseases, etc., there is much to support the realization that physicians are only human. Have you ever heard of a physician telling a paraplegic to rise up and walk? Well, this is what the fisherman Peter said to the lame man at the gate of the Temple. He simply said, "In the name of Jesus Christ the

Nazarene—walk!" (Acts 3:6). Note that the command was made *in* the name of Jesus Christ. And the man leaped up, stood and walked. The orthopedic specialist would soon be a nonentity if this were repeated in our day. Contemplate this fact: handkerchiefs and aprons brought into contact with the apostle Paul healed the people of various diseases and even evil spirits departed (see Acts 19:11,12).

The medical men and women of our day, although backed by many technological skills and much experience, are still novices in the art of healing and in the mysteries of the internal body. They are traveling a dark tunnel with many twists and turns. Even the greatest surgeons and internists are specialists in the sense that they know only a great deal about very little. But this is to be expected as they are not the creators of the most marvelous machine in the world—the human body. At best, they are willing apprentices (we hope) to be taught by the Great Physician.

It is amazing how man uses his common sense when it comes to taking care of machines and equipment and yet is so ignorant and helpless when it comes to the care of his body. He will avidly read the instruction manual for maintenance and repair of his automobile and considers it high treason to turn it over to just any service station mechanic. Yet when his body machinery is sluggish or malfunctioning, he knows only to turn to the physician and druggist for care. The human body is the most intricate machine in the universe and we must take care that we do not subject it indiscriminately to any and all who declare themselves to be physicians. This is not to advocate that medical science and physicians are to be shunned, but it is to recognize that the knowledge and skill they have is only miniscule.

God encased the internal organs of our bodies in skin—like the locked hood of the Rolls-Royce. He didn't intend for anyone to get in and tamper with them. What cannot be absorbed through the skin must be inserted by a needle. Or an incision has to be made in the skin. (The gastrointestinal tract is only a continuation of the outer skin that we see.) And when a surgeon performs an operation he is tampering with an internal system which God intended should not be tampered with. But, you ask, don't surgeons remove diseased or injured organs or parts of the body, or growths such as tumors, that are detrimental to the body? Of course. But after such traumatic episodes the body heals itself. These surgical actions help the body to recover but healing, in itself, is not due to the surgery.

Although God has "locked the hood" to our internal system, He has not left us without responsibility in the care of it. We cannot eat, drink and play without restraint.

Healthful living includes moderation in eating, drinking and resting. We need daily exercise, fresh air, sunshine, cleanliness and proper hygiene of our bodies and our surroundings.

We must strive for positive mental and emotional attitudes. In fact mental health is sadly neglected in this day and age when it is most urgently needed. Did you know that psychiatrists have the highest suicide rate among physicians? Yet these are the very specialists trained to care for those with mental problems! Better mental therapy is found in Psalm 37. No one can give guidelines for rest, diet, exercise, etc., but each man is monitored by the Spirit of God dwelling in him who will instruct him as to what is right and wrong and what is adequate of the right. Healthful living is not the responsibility of the government and science. It is your personal responsibility.

Therefore, the outlook for the 1980s and beyond is that we are responsible health-carers with our locked hoods under the care of God. But it takes great faith and discipline to leave your complete living in the hands of God. May you have faith to do so.

2

ARE YOU A HYPOCHONDRIAC?

by Audrey Carli

Janet, age 48, heard her neighbor describing the agonizing pain involved with her kidney stone. Janet had been feeling pain in her bladder area recently. She wondered if she too had kidney stones. Finally, she went to the doctor. A urine specimen was studied. Janet's illness: an acute urinary infection. "Quite a difference between treating that and having to undergo surgery to remove kidney stones, Janet," the doctor said.

"I should have come in for an examination sooner. My mind really played tricks on me. I was sure I'd need kidney stone surgery."

In another case, John, age 48, developed pain in his knuckles. It was so severe he knew he was getting arthritis. His wife Marlis had had arthritis for several years. She developed it in her late thirties. John empathized when he saw Marlis wince with pain when her medication was wearing off. He wished he could bear her arthritic pain. Now both would suffer from the disease. But the doctor examined John and said he had no sign of arthritis. "You have so much sympathy for your wife, you have imagined having arthritis. It has happened before. Some men feel pain when their wives are in childbirth labor. They so want to share the pain, they actually feel pain. But it's really in the mind."

This problem is sometimes termed hypochondria. The experts tell us what hypochondria is. Those who have overcome this problem tell us how they did it.

Hypochondria is an obsessive preoccupation with one's body or a bodily organ or with health in general. The word refers to a portion of the upper abdomen once thought to be the source of all illness, the parts under the cartilage of the breastbone.

The hypochondriac's psychosomatic symptoms may be as gripping as gunshot wounds. But they may evolve so that he actually feels genuine chest pains, severe migraine headaches, asthmatic wheezing, or laryngitis. Or he may develop other symptoms.

How often does hypochondria strike? Some health experts estimate that as many as 75 percent of patients visiting doctors have nothing physically wrong. Ten years ago a Mayo Clinic (Rochester, Minnesota) division study concluded that 50 to 55 percent of symptoms reported were not based on specific diseases. "At least half the patients here [have problems] not due to disease, per se, but to other factors related to anxiety, fatigue, concern, stress, pressure," said Dr. Earl T. Carter, professor of preventive medicine at Mayo Clinic. "Are we going to call all of them hypochondriacs? No. By that definition, we'd all be."

In reality, millions of healthy people suspect that they are ill. It is often a temporary reaction to stress—such as the worry many suffered after the Three Mile Island nuclear plant leak. After that occurrence, it was reported that hundreds who feared radiation exposure visited doctors complaining of skin rashes and a barrage of likely symptoms. Many medical students develop illness symptoms after studying about a certain disease.

If the symptoms can be dealt with as simple hypochondria brought on by an understandable worry source, life can again be peaceful for the victims. However, if symptoms continue, hypochondria becomes a threat. Emotional anxiety and depression may result. Unneeded medical care may follow.

Another big reason hypochondria strikes is because a person feels lonely. The victim may need affection and someone to care. "Anyone learns by being ill that you get some degree of affection, caring," said Benjamin Belden, executive director of the Chicago Center for Behavior Modification.

Some lonely persons with hypochondria are expressing a need to be mothered, said Dr. Maria Piers, distinguished service professor at Erikson Institute. "This person takes overly good care of himself because [he feels] nobody else does."

One woman who kept thinking she had a disease finally went to a doctor who was known to listen to his patients' problems. He was the type who had empathy and the patient felt cared for. The doctor listened to the patient's symptoms and as the woman talked, she revealed she had worried for years she would get cancer as did her mother and grandmother. Regular physical exams showed she did not have cancer. The doctor's sympathetic listening *and* the physical examination helped her overcome her deep fear of getting cancer.

Others who feel overly concerned about having an illness, even though the doctor (several in some cases) said there was no evidence of disease, need to find ways to forget about the illness worry. One man who became worried about heart disease after several friends in his age group died from heart attacks had a complete physical examination three times in one year at three different clinics. Each time he was found in excellent physical condition. The last doctor told him, "It's understandable that you are concerned about your heart. One of my good friends died suddenly from a heart attack. We were friends since boyhood. It stunned me. I'm a doctor and I felt the need for a thorough physical examination too. I was relieved to learn all's well. It's the same with you. Get busy with a hobby. Get your mind off yourself. That's the advice I gave myself. I give you the same advice."

That man enrolled in an adult night class at the local high school. He made a bookcase, picnic table and other items in the woodwork course. He got so engrossed in his hobby, he forgot about his worry over possible heart trouble. "I also made sure I ate the proper diet for a healthy heart—one low in fat. I walked two or more miles daily. And the woodwork relieved the stress that was making my heart pound at times, giving me heart-disease fear. I feel great since I started my hobby. I advise getting a hobby to everyone with worries on his or her mind."

A woman who was given a clean bill of health, even though she worried about having something wrong with her head because of frequent headaches, was told to get a job. She had told the doctor she had too many hours to think now that her children were grown and had left home. "That job made me get involved with other things and forget myself. No longer did I regret not having more housework and more child tending to do. I became a nurse's aide in a hospital. I get inner peace in helping others. I feel healthier than in years. The headaches faded when my job started. Now I realize I'd been under stress because of my life change after the children grew up."

Another woman who had been busy all her life raising a family, then working at a job, and finally retiring, said she developed all sorts of ailments when she had so many hours and not much to do with them. "My husband kept busy with church activities with the men. The women were not as active. I felt sick but didn't know how to explain my symptoms. So I had a complete physical. Nothing was wrong. The doctor told me I'd earned my free time. He emphasized, 'Take time to smell the roses of life.'

"Now I walk to the river curling through our property. I feel joy in seeing the sunbeams dance on the water in silvery shimmers. I want to join the birds in song as they chirp as if glad for the blessing of another day. I take time to smell the roses and other flowers. I sniff the clean air after a rain.

"There are so many things to see, smell and hear in nature. I'm thankful for my free time now. I can squeeze the joy out of life and be glad I've learned to appreciate all the blessings. My advice is to take time to 'smell the roses in life' no matter what your age. I count my daily blessings and . . . worry over that pain here or there is soon forgotten. We all have a pain now and then. If the doctor says there is no illness, I'll believe. I can always get a second opinion. But I'll make sure to take time daily to enjoy life— and to 'smell the roses.' "

Hypochondria can plague you with illness fears. But if the doctor(s) tells you all is well, enjoy life and glory in daily blessings—as you take time to smell the roses.

3

MENTAL HURDLES OF LIFE

by Dr. John R. Cheydleur

In Fullerton, California, a sprightly woman in her mid-eighties spends every other week "house-sitting" for couples who are on vacation. Periodically she is visited by attentive young women who roomed with her 10 years ago as college students, when she was running a boarding house in her active seventies. Her poise, good humor, and sense of purpose show that she is winning the race of life.

One of the young women visiting her, a medical receptionist, shared with me the joy and radiance which had been brought into her life by this graceful, active person. She also shared her experience with a man in his early nineties, a visitor to her medical clinic in Florida. This man is also active, but rather than being full of sweetness and light, he is full of vinegar and anger! It is not uncommon for him to pick up the magazines on the reception room coffee table and throw them across the room in exasperation, if asked to do something which he does not like.

What is the secret of activity into later life which these two very different people possess? What makes them different? What can you and I learn from their lives and the lives of others that would help us move into successive stages of maturity with confidence and a measure of success?

Father Charles Curran, Ph.D., famous priest-psychologist and former head of the American Catholic Psychological Association, says that in persons of extreme age he finds there to be only two attitudes toward life. One attitude is that of profound gratitude for the goodness of life. The other is anger and ingratitude and a feeling of having been cheated by life.

There is also a third response to life, a response which Dr. Curran did not note because it is less common among those who survive than among those who die at an earlier age. This attitude is that of passive resignation, a kind of fatalism that says life is not good and I can't win against it either. Unlike active acceptance of life or active anger and challenge to life, this attitude is rather like that of the small boy on the playground in the midst of a fight who cries, "Uncle!" Then, after being released from his opponent's hold he just lies on the ground and refuses to get up and rejoin the swirling hordes of children on the playground. Some adults are like this boy. They have simply curled up to die, lying down between the sixteenth and seventeenth hurdles in the race—refusing to rejoin the excitement and challenge of living.

The famous psycho-social theorist, Erik H. Erikson, has noted that there are eight stages in life, each of which, if successfully mastered, creates a mindset which helps us to be successful in completing the continuing tasks which will come in the next stage of life. The apostle Paul also likened his own life to a race: "I press on toward the goal for the prize of the upward call of God in Christ Jesus (Phil. 3:14).

As we trace the stages in the race of life, we will also note the mental hurdles which are involved at each stage. Ask yourself which of these hurdles have been successfully crossed in your own life, and which of them are still to be crossed on the way to the finish line.

The first hurdle in your life occurred between birth and the age of eight months. The task which psychologists attach to this stage is entitled, "Establishing Object Constancy," which is a fancy way of saying that we need *to believe that our mother or other loving parent object still exists even when out of our sight and hearing.* Crossing this hurdle successfully sets up a basic trust towards life, while failing to cross it sets up a basic mistrust which can poison all our relationships.

If you tripped (or were tripped!) crossing this hurdle, you find it difficult to build trust relationships with other people and even with God. You have yet to learn the security of the psalmist who says, "God is my helper! He is a friend of mine!" (Ps. 54:4, *TLB*).

The second hurdle in your life appeared during the period between 18 months and three years. During this stage the task is that of *learning self-control and limit-setting without developing shame and doubt.*

Contemporary research suggests that the primary influence in successfully leaping this particular hurdle is a positive, but firm, parental atmosphere.

The poised, self-assured, ulcer-free person who has successfully crossed this hurdle is contrasted with the dissipated sales manager who has never learned self-control and the overscrupulous librarian who is unable to believe that anything she does is acceptable.

The third stage of life, beginning in the three- to six-year-old period, lays the foundation for the development of a conscience, and for a pro-active attitude about exploring and meeting the challenge of the world around us. The mental hurdle to be negotiated at this stage is that of *being able to let go of some of our dependence upon our parents and reaching out to build relationships with our peers.*

Just as you can think of many examples of adults who have not yet successfully jumped the hurdle of stage two, and are therefore either unwilling to live with the necessary moral limits on their own behavior, or who have fallen off the other side of this hurdle and are constantly looking over their shoulders wondering if every least little act is in some way going to be offensive to another person or to divine authority, you will be able to look at yourself and other persons and note those situations which show that hurdle number three has yet to be successfully crossed.

The "company man" who maintains a good relationship with his superiors but refuses to become socially involved with other persons may never have jumped this hurdle. Likewise, your own overdependence on the security aspects of a job, inhibiting your desire to be creative and to reach out to further fields, may also be traced to the need to cross this particular mental hurdle.

The fourth hurdle, which first presents itself between ages 6 and 12, is, perhaps, a little taller than the hurdles which have come before. Crossing this hurdle may be dependent upon the successful crossing of the previous barriers. The mental hurdle involved here is that of *achieving a sense of one's own ability as a contributing worker, rather than feeling that one is inferior and incapable*. This sense of industry is gained from those things which one's *peer group approves*, such as prowess in baseball, playground games, or other group activities of youth culture. However, even the person of high intrinsic ability may not complete this hurdle at this time if the ability which he or she has is a type which is not important to his or her peer culture during this age period.

You may be a brilliant person, a person who has the capacity to be a tremendous contributor to society, but you may be limiting your own contribution through a pervading sense of inferiority which is due to your need to hurdle this leftover fence in life's road.

While some persons develop a sense of discouragement during this period, others emerge from this stage with a supreme sense of self-confidence about their ability to contribute to life. Alfred Adler's compensation theory suggests that there may also be a third class of persons, those who develop a tremendous sense of anger, challenge, and an "I'll-prove-that-I'm-as-good-as-any-of-them!" attitude. One such man, responding to a health study questionnaire, wrote in his own answer to one question: "I don't *get* ulcers; I *give* ulcers!"

The fifth stage in the life cycle is the one which you probably remember most clearly. This stage, adolescence, occurs between the ages of 12 and 18. If the earlier hurdles have already been successfully negotiated, the task to be faced during this stage is *the development of a personal ego identity*. The accrued confidence which we have developed from successfully completing the earlier stages allows us to work through the role confusions of adolescence and emerge with a clear self-identity.

This is the theory. However, in American society we do not become confident about our abilities as workers until sometime during the teenage years so that this next hurdle becomes one to be jumped during the early twenties, rather than during the traditional adolescent period. It is not uncommon in today's society to see many young adults, even into their late twenties, whose sense of self-identity has not come together in a way which would indicate that they have successfully crossed this hurdle.

During the period of the twenties, the sixth hurdle appears on the track. As the task of self-identity moves toward resolution, we are also faced with the mental hurdle of *learning to fuse our own clear identity with the clear identity of another person or persons*. This task takes its most intimate and permanent form in marriage, but is also present in religious affiliation, the development of work groups, and the building of lasting personal relationships.

The difficulty for many persons in crossing this hurdle is that the prior hurdle of developing self-identity has not yet been crossed. We are then faced with the paradox of trying to merge two fuzzy identities together, with the risk that this premature merger may inhibit the development of a clear sense of self—necessary for a successful merger. The result is a tragic series of divorces and other broken relationships, occurring because we have tried to merge identities which did not yet exist in concrete form.

You may be one of those persons who, even in later life, have still not crossed this hurdle of developing intimacy instead of isolation because you approached this hurdle at an earlier age when your own identity was not yet developed and found that you were not ready to successfully negotiate it at that time. Now in later life your identity has become more clear, but you are afraid to take another run at this very important hurdle in self-development. It should be noted that I am not advocating here the loss of your own self-identity, but rather the fusing of two clearly defined identities, a fusing which cannot be clearly and successfully completed without your own personal self-awareness.

For the person who has successfully (and possibly miraculously!) negotiated the previous six hurdles by age 30, the seventh hurdle pops up out of the ground to be crossed during the next 10 to 20 years. As you become aware of the arrival and growth of your own offspring or of the children of your peers, you are faced with a new task. This is the task of *passing on what you know and have learned to the next generation*. Successful negotiation of this hurdle may take many forms. It may occur in child rearing, the most traditional and continuing task of society. It may occur in teaching or in writing articles such as this one.

For my father, Benjamin Cheydleur, it meant moving out of a lucrative career in commercial computer design to the teaching of his principles to young doctoral-level computer engineers.

The person who bangs his leg on this hurdle and fails to cross it becomes the person whose most obvious attribute is that of "I don't care." Both the person who is grateful to life and the person who continues to dare life in an angry fashion will find some way to pass on their philosophy and life experiences to others. The person who fails to take up this challenge, the challenge of communicating to and establishing the next generation, is most likely to become a statistic rather than a live person by the time he or she should have reached age 75 or 80.

All of us are familiar with the person who takes "early retirement" at age 35 or 40 with a sense of hopelessness and a feeling that he or she has nothing to contribute to the future. The difference is not always tied to the nature of your vocation, for some persons in very simple jobs are able to feel a profound sense of being able to pass on wisdom to the younger persons around them. On a positive note, some people break through their sense of frustration about not being able to contribute to life by becoming involved in mid-life career changes and redirection of goals.

The psalmist recalls his own reaching out to God for help in crossing this hurdle when, after crying out about being "knocked . . . to the ground" and "paralyzed with fear," he asks, "Show me where to walk, for my prayer is sincere" (Ps. 143:3,4,8 *TLB*).

The eighth and final stage of the life cycle, one which we saw so successfully achieved by the woman described at the beginning of this article, is that of *developing ego integrity instead of despair*. In this stage, the hurdle is successfully mastered by achieving a sense of emotional integrity, a sense of spiritual fellowship with one's Creator, and the acceptance of the responsibility of one's position in life. One writer has called this the development of "a comradeship with the ordering of distant times and orders of events."

The passive person, the one who gives up early, probably never even gets close enough to see this hurdle. The angry, challenging person may possess enough vinegar to get in sight of it, but vinegar is not the secret of a peaceful, well-integrated personality, prepared to continue in active service for many years and equally prepared for a calm transition through death and into that which lies beyond this life.

The race of life has very simple rules. Each of the eight hurdles must be crossed as it appears. All skipped hurdles must be made up in some way. Then as you and I cross life's hurdles, one-by-one, and rejoice that we have come far enough to discover the next hurdle on the track, we can look together toward the time when we will be able to say with Paul, "I have finished the course, I have kept the faith; in the future there is laid up for me the crown of righteousness" (2 Tim. 4:7,8, *TLB*).

4

HOW TO ESCAPE THE DISCOURAGEMENT TRAP

by Dr. John R. Cheydleur

"Have you ever heard about the devil's garage sale?" My publisher, Bob Smith, posed this question for me as we discussed this article for *Total Health* magazine. This is the story:

All the sub-demons and junior devils came to the devil's garage sale to buy up assorted instruments of torture which the devil no longer personally needed.

Thumbscrews tagged "guilt" were a popular item. A giant rubber mallet named "nagging" was sold quickly. The bidding was fast and furious for several sets of spiked chains labeled "addiction." The various whips, maces and sundry other tortures were sold until only one item remained.

Over in one corner of the garage a small item stood by itself on a table, covered by a cloth, with the legend "Not For Sale" scribbled on a ragged sheet of paper next to it.

The sub-demons and junior devils had been trying all day to find out what was under the cloth, and more than one had had his hand slapped or his tail twisted for trying to look under the cloth.

Now only the covered item remained. The devil went over to it saying, "This is my most powerful weapon. I will never sell it!" So saying, he lifted the cloth to reveal a slender wedge, obviously worn from much use. He held it up proudly and said, "When nothing else works, I just find a small crack and tap in this wedge—its name is DISCOURAGE-MENT."

Discouragement can sneak up on you. Often it seems to appear without warning, even when many parts of your life seem to be satisfactory or even positive. Contrary to the way it seems, discouragement has clear-cut, well-researched causes. You can identify the potential or actual causes of discouragement in your life. By tackling the *causes* of discouragement, rather than allowing yourself to be subjected to the feelings of self-doubt and energy loss which discouragement produces, you can get out of the discouragement trap.

If you are feeling the curse of discouragement it may seem that nothing can change your fate. However, the Scripture reminds us that "A curse without cause does not alight" (Prov. 26:2) so that, as the causes are dealt with, the discouragement will be eliminated.

The reason that so much well-meaning advice does not help when a person feels discouragement is that most such advice is designed to be "encouraging." The problem with attempting to use "encouragement" is that *these are not opposite ends of the same spectrum*. Dr. Frederick Herzberg has performed extensive research proving that "encourage-ment" and "discouragement" are composed of totally different factors.

The six encouragement factors documented by Dr. Herzberg are: (1) achievement; (2) recognition; (3) a satisfying task; (4) personal responsibility; (5) a chance for advancement; (6) opportunity for personal growth. When one or more of these factors are operating a person feels "encouraged," good about himself or herself, pleased with life.

However, *it is possible to be both encouraged and discouraged at the same time*. There are 10 factors which, taken singly or together, can create a sense of discouragement, making you doubt your own self-worth, lose vital energy necessary to perform even ordinary tasks, and feel "trapped" with no way out. While it is vitally important for us to be "encouraged," it is even more basic that we not be "discouraged."

I have divided the 10 discouragement factors into three life areas on the accompanying "Discouragement Inventory." The "Discouragement Inventory" will give you a basic discouragement rating. If you score higher than four on any one factor, or higher than 28 overall, it is important that you examine the area(s) of difficulty and do some concrete planning for changes, either by yourself or with a trusted friend or counselor. Remember that *discouragement does not "just happen." It is caused, and when you change the cause, you will change the result*.

Discouragement is indeed a subtle wedge, one which has crippled many a runner in the race of life. As you identify and eliminate the causes of discouragement in your life you become free to move into areas of positive action and progress so that you will be able to say, along with St. Paul, "I have fought the good fight, I have finished the course" (2 Tim. 4:7)

THE DISCOURAGEMENT INVENTORY

Circle the number from 1 to 5 which best describes your current or immediate past situation in relation to each factor. Score 1 if no problem exists; score 5 for an area of major difficulty. Add your total score at the bottom.

No Problem—Major Problem   **Area One—Power Relationship**

1   2   3   4   5   1. Poor supervision from boss, teacher or other authority figure.

1   2   3   4   5   2. Poor relationship with authority figure (boss, spouse, parent, church or social leader).

1   2   3   4   5   3. Unfair or predictable policy administration from boss or authority figure.

1   2   3   4   5   4. Unhappy relationships with subordinates (job or family).

Area Two—Security and Comfort

1 2 3 4 5   5. Inadequate, unsafe, or unsanitary conditions at work or at home.

1 2 3 4 5   6. Inadequate financial arrangements (salary, allowance, budget).

1 2 3 4 5   7. Lack of job security or family stability.

Area Three—Personal

1 2 3 4 5   8. Lack of status, reputation (vocational or social).

1 2 3 4 5   9. Poor peer relationships (job, social, family).

1 2 3 4 5   10. Difficulties in personal life (family relationships, personal habits, guilt).

TOTAL _____

Ratings: 10-17   You are more free than most people.
18-28   Normal range. Plan to change areas which scored 4 or 5.
29-40   High stress. Tackle each factor separately. Do not punish yourself.
41-50   You need a friend. See a good counselor.

Based on the original research of Frederick Herzberg, "Motivation and Hygiene Factors."

5

THE SECRET OF SELF-AFFIRMATION

by Dr. John R. Cheydleur

"I want to feel self-affirmed, but more times than I'd like to admit, I feel defeated and depressed."

Have you said or thought these words? Do you try to be a self-affirming person but find that your attempts to think positively only work part of the time? You are not alone.

My friend, Sam Spadero, is an incredibly self-affirming man, one of the most successful account executives in 3M's Com Systems Division. After a tragic auto accident two-and-a-half years ago Sam became a Christian, changed his life-style, and began to claim success and prosperity in his life on the basis of God's promises. This worked magnificently, but there were perplexing exceptions. "I know this business of confessing positive ideas before God works, but I feel like something funny occurs when I tell people about a sale that I'm sure God is going to give me, and then it falls through."

Have you ever felt like my friend Sam? There is a secret to effective self-affirmation which can make all the difference in the world. In order to understand that secret, let's take a moment to comprehend the opposite of self-affirmation, which is depression.

Dr. Robert Pfeiler, M.D., formerly director of Community Mental Health for the State of Minnesota, and now supervising psychiatrist for the California Christian Institute in Orange County, California, says that, "Depression is caused by the emotions of anger and hate being 'introjected' or turned inward." People who express their anger and hate openly may be unpleasant persons to be around, but they rarely get ulcers or other psychosomatic illnesses associated with depression.

We most often become depressed when we are angry but cannot or do not express our emotions, thus allowing those negative emotions to turn in on ourselves. I recently surveyed children waiting in a theater line to see the film "The Empire Strikes Back" and received some very revealing answers to the question, "What makes you depressed?"

Among the children's responses were: When I spill my ice cream; when I fight with my brother; when my father and mother argue; when I get a B- for a grade; when I have a cold; when other kids get new things that I don't have; when I can't find a pair of socks.

As each of the small angers and hates builds up, neither being expressed nor being resolved through true forgiveness and reconciliation, these are pushed down into the subconscious mind, creating a negative emotional pool which emerges as depression, lethargy and a feeling of worthlessness.

In much the same way, the first step in gaining a sense of self-affirmation and self-worth comes through understanding and experiencing the emotions of love and joy. This is the *"secret" of effective self-affirmation*. Just as we do not program ourselves for depression by dwelling on despair but by turning the emotions of hate and anger inward upon ourselves, we cannot program self-affirmation simply by meditating on positive thoughts, as valuable as that exercise is. We must find a way to turn the emotions of love and joy inward to create a positive emotional pool which will express itself in feelings of self-affirmation and self-worth.

My friend Sam Spadero has typed up a copy of the most powerful love chapter in the Bible (1 Corinthians 13) and carries it with him to meditate upon. He says, "It's strange, John, but the more I meditate on love and ask God to make me a really loving person, the more successful and confident I become."

The reason is simple: *as hate and anger turned inward make us feel worthless and depressed, their opposites, love and joy, make us feel self-affirming and confident.*

The group of children which we surveyed said that they experienced self-affirmation in a variety of ways tied to love and joy: When I'm eating the things I like; when I do puppet shows in front of an audience; when I run races; when I play the piano when no one's telling me; when my team is winning a baseball game; when I'm singing.

There is a powerful second step to the self-affirmation secret which must also be grasped. Just as superficially-expressed anger and hate may do damage to the world around us but do not become turned inward to create depression, our superficial expressions of positive emotions such as love, joy and confidence may make the world around us happier but do not become turned inward to create a sense of self-affirmation and self-worth.

Every poised woman knows that the way she feels about the way she looks often has more to do with her elegant underwear, which no one else sees, than with her well-made dress or carefully-tailored pantsuit. Recently a men's underwear manufacturer has picked up this same theme through an ad in which a man riding an elevator exclaims, "I feel good all under!"

Jesus taught that we should allow the positive emotions of faith, hope and love to grow and deepen within us. "When you pray, go into your inner room, and when you have shut your door, pray to your Father who is in secret, and your Father who sees in secret will repay you" (Matt. 6:6).

The spiritual and psychological thrust of this teaching is that love and joy should be held on to and allowed to grow. Often our temptation is to try to get others to affirm our positive emotions (and to reconcile our own doubts) rather than to develop a deepening sense of confidence and faith between us and a loving heavenly Father.

Of course it is important to interact with other people, but the source of our positive feelings about ourselves cannot be the affirmation of others. Instead, the source of our confidence must be the powerful secret affirmation, a self-affirmation which springs out of a positive emotional pool created by the continuous infusion of love and joy through positive personal experiences like those named by the children we interviewed, and through a continuous love life with God Himself.

How can you do this? First, take a simple sheet of paper and make column headings: **LOVE** and **JOY.** Then, under each heading, list the activities and experiences in which you have experienced love or affirmed your abilities. List activities which created these positive emotions for you. Include at least 10 items under each heading. You might be surprised to find how many good things you could be experiencing more often!

Next, locate the book that has more psychological helps in it than any reference publication you can buy, the Bible. *Underline at least 10 passages which make you feel joyful, loving or loved.* (Some powerful passages can be found in Psalms 23; 46; and 91; as well as 1 Corinthians 13; Galatians 5:23; 1 John 4.)

Without getting tied up in complicated tables and charts, make it a point to experience something on your list and/or to meditate upon a love- or joy-focused Scripture portion every day. Imagine what even one telephone call to someone you love or one small friendly comment to a child could do to make you feel good.

When you regularly program yourself to do those things which make you experience the emotions of love and joy, no matter how you feel at the time you initiate these activities, you change yourself in a powerful way.

As you maintain this simple program you will be feeding your subconscious and developing a pool of positive emotions from which your sense of self-affirmation and self-worth will grow.

6

REFLECTIONS ON GROWING OLD

by Herbert A. De Souza, S.J.

The only reason why most of us consent to growing old is that the alternative is even more depressing. But we know only too well the attendants of old age: waning powers, crippling disabilities, humiliating dependence, isolation from life's mainstream, and worst of all, loneliness, rejection, oblivion. Living death, some have actually called it.

How could anyone as intelligent as Browning, one of the foremost poets of the last century, and an aging widower with poignant memories of an incredibly happy marriage, ever come to pen lines like these?

> Grow old with me;
> The best is yet to be,
> The last of life for which the
>   first was made.

Romantic he certainly was; naive he certainly was not. Those who knew him intimately bore testimony to his great courage and unabating optimism in his sunset years, and an even more abundant manifestation of these qualities as he faced death: "One fight more, the last and the best!"

His secret? Well, nothing secret about it really. From antiquity men and women have discovered that it is not *what* you face in old age that is important, but *how* you face it. Grasp the nettle, and it ceases to sting. The old Roman philosopher Seneca expressed it well: "Let us cherish and love old age, for it is full of pleasures *if we know how to use it.*" Browning's contemporary and friend Lord Tennyson recalls for us in his *Ulysses* the philosophy of that great Greek hero of the Trojan war: "Old age gives more than it takes away."

What it takes away we know all too well. What it gives needs recurrent recall.

First and foremost it gives us leisure to do the things we always claimed we wanted to do but protested we couldn't because of the more urgent demands of earning a living, supporting a family, fulfilling responsibilities to parents, relatives, friends, colleagues, church, organizations we belonged to—the list was endless; our precious moments of leisure all frittered away. Like the character in T.S. Eliot's poem, we "measured out our life in coffee spoons."

In his illuminating study of American mores, *Of Time, Work & Leisure,* political scientist Sebastian de Grazia writes: "There is no doubt that Americans have reached a new level of life. Whether it is a good life is another matter. This much is clear: it is a life without leisure . . . Leisure is a state of being free of everyday necessity, and the activities of leisure are those one would engage in for their own sake. As fact or ideal, it is rarely approached in the industrial world."

Now, in old age, leisure is all we have, and our salvation lies in learning how to use it, how to profit by it, how to be so absorbed in it that we forget that aging, ailing aching body of ours.

For many, the reading of books achieves this best; not

just novels, but history, science, philosophy, religion. Reading keeps the mind active, and as the Romans discovered long ago, *mens sana in corpore sano*—a healthy mind makes for a healthy body.

Some, alas, find their eyes unequal to the task. The great English poet Milton was such a one; when he lost his eyesight his first complaint, as he expressed it so movingly in a sonnet, *On His Blindness*, was that his "one talent which was death to hide was lodged with him useless." Then he recalled that God didn't really need his talents, only his self-importance had deluded him into thinking so. God has all the angels in heaven to do His bidding. Our task here below is to tune our wills to His:

> They also serve who only
>   stand and wait.

But Milton found something to do while he was standing and waiting. He wrote his masterpiece, *Paradise Lost*. When Beethoven went deaf, he pressed his knees against the piano to pick up its vibrations and wrote some of his greatest symphonies, including the immortal Ninth. There is always something we can do if we really want to do it. If lemons are all we are left with, we can let them sour us or we can make lemonade for our thirsty friends.

Then there are hobbies we can cultivate. America offers more opportunities for these, and more centers and instructors for the cultivation of them, than any country on earth. Any hobby will do: stamps, carpentry, gardening, crossword puzzles, painting (remember Grandma Moses at 90?), needlepoint (no, Rosie Grier was not an old lady), macrame, writing—letters, poetry, family history, childhood reminiscences, life in the old country, life on the farm, life in the small town before it became the oversize city it is now. If writing does not come easy, a tape recorder is God's answer to arthritis.

Perhaps the greatest achievement of old age is a philosophy of life. We thought we had one, but that was mainly for export. It is only when old age forced us to apply it to ourselves that we realized how empty it was. "There never was a philosopher," wrote Shakespeare, "who could bear the toothache patiently."

Now, Bible in hand, we can forge a philosophy out of the matched experience of our lives with those tried and true philosophies of the men of God in the Bible: Abraham, Jacob, Job, Joseph, Gideon, David, Samuel, and Christ Himself. The women of the Bible are no less inspiring: Sara, Rachel, Anna, Hannah, Esther, the mother of Christ, Eunice and Lois. What these men and women have to teach us is, above all else, faith and trust in God when everything around seems to crumble. The twenty-third Psalm says it all: "Though I walk through the valley of the shadow of death, I fear no evil; for Thou art with me" (v. 4).

This is indeed the full life, the graceful life, for it is a life full of grace. And when it draws to a close, as draw it must, we can say with that great poet philosopher Walter Savage Landor:

I have warmed my hands at
    the fire of life;
It dies, and I am ready to
    depart.

7

WHAT YOUR SLEEP HABITS MAY BE SAYING ABOUT YOUR PERSONALITY

by Robin Tracy

Psychologists say that the way you sit, stand and dress may reveal your personality. Now the experts tell us that our sleep habits also reveal personality traits.

M.W. Johns, a sleep researcher at Monash University in Melbourne, Australia, asked 104 medical students to fill out questionnaires about their sleep habits, and then had each student take a personality test.

Johns found that students who had a lot of difficulty falling asleep were almost always worriers. The personality tests revealed that they had more anxiety and a lower sense of self-esteem than their peers, reports the Better Sleep Council, an organization that gives out information on sleep and sleep research.

Students who reported waking up frequently during the night turned out to be the ones who repressed their problems, according to the personality tests, and who had trouble admitting to any difficulties in their interpersonal relationships.

The students who awakened frequently also reported more physical symptoms, feelings of weakness or dizziness, than their peers. The researchers hypothesized that the emotional problems which they couldn't talk about were emerging as physical symptoms.

The worriers, by contrast, who could talk freely about their anxieties even though they kept them from falling asleep easily, did not have many physical complaints.

Does getting to sleep very easily mean you have everything under control? Not necessarily. Johns found that people who get to sleep unusually quickly also tend to wake up frequently during the night and were, once again, people who repress their problems.

Because they have little on their conscious minds, they have little trouble falling asleep, he reasoned. But once asleep their defenses weaken and problems come to the surface, causing them to awaken.

One result of frequent awakening is that a person doesn't get as much sleep as he or she needs. As a result, people who awaken frequently take more naps during the day than most people, trying to make up for the sleep they didn't get at night.

Johns also seems to have proven the old adage about the early bird getting the worm. Johns found that early risers get better grades than late risers (who got up an average of 42 minutes later, both during the week and on weekends).

The early risers slept better, too—73 percent reported that their sleep was "very good." The late risers by comparison did less well on their examinations, and only 40 percent reported that their sleep was "very good."

There were also differences in personality between the two groups. The early risers were conscientious and had a realistic self-image, while the late risers were unrealistic about their capabilities and limitations and tended to be more rebellious and unconventional.

Another study comparing good and poor sleepers showed not only that good sleepers have better psychological profiles than poor sleepers, but that there are physiological differences too. The central nervous system was more highly active in the poor sleepers than in the good sleepers, both when awake and asleep.

Johns concluded that detailed descriptions of sleep habits provide reliable information about a person's psychological make-up, taking into account, of course, the person's age and any physical illness.

But what does all this mean to you if you're a worrier who has trouble falling asleep, or if your problems wake you up at night? It may merely mean that you have a lot on your mind and that your problems are interfering with your sleep.

You might want to talk things over with a friend or seek some professional help such as counseling at a sleep clinic, but in the meantime the Better Sleep Council recommends that you don't do anything else to interfere with your already troubled sleep.

- Don't drink tea or coffee shortly before going to bed. The caffeine can keep you awake.
- Don't drink alcohol. Heavy drinking may "knock you out," but when the alcohol wears off, there is a tendency to wake up.
- Make sure your room is dark and quiet. Both undue noise and light can interfere with your rest.

8

HOW TO HANDLE ANXIETY

by Marion Wells

The frequency with which people are turning to tranquilizers to calm down has a number of health professionals
rather uptight.

An estimated *five billion tranquilizer pills* are prescribed in the U.S. each year. Top FDA officials, among
others, are worried that too many Americans are turning too
quickly to chemicals for comfort.

Such drugs may have their emergency uses in helping
people through a crisis or mental or emotional illness, but
reaching for them routinely to deal with the stresses of daily
living is another matter. People who become too reliant on
chemicals to cope could wind up having worse problems
coping with the chemicals, experts say. Among the risks
they may face are physical or psychological dependency, or
both, a serious withdrawal syndrome, and the dangers of
drug interactions.

Concern centers on the so-called "minor tranquilizers,"
also called anxiolytics for their use in treating "anxiety."
Numbered among them is "the most frequently prescribed
drug in the United States," diazepam (brand name Valium),

one of the benzodiazepines. Such drugs are different from the "major tranquilizers," a whole separate class of medications used to treat psychotic disorders such as schizophrenia.

Effectiveness of the minor tranquilizers over the long term (more than four months) "has not been assessed by systematic clinical studies," says the FDA. They also say that people who use the drugs in high doses for long periods run the highest risk of getting hooked on the chemicals.

Physical dependence, authorities say, may result in withdrawal symptoms, some of which may include "agitation, insomnia, sweating, tremors, abdominal and muscle cramps, vomiting." An insidious aspect is that such symptoms may be similar to those that triggered the use of tranquilizers in the first place, making people think they still need the drugs. And experts caution that people should get their physician's help in getting off tranquilizers so they can be medically monitored to minimize any hazards.

Another concern experts have is psychological dependence. Turning on to tranquilizers to tone down stress may turn off the search for other ways of coping, they fear. They point out that pills don't solve problems, they just *temporarily* ease symptoms.

Minor tranquilizers act as central nervous system depressants. They can interact with a variety of other drugs, including the nation's number one nonprescription drug, alcohol. A recent FDA Drug Bulletin noted findings from the Drug Abuse Warning Network (DAWN) for 1980. The country's most popular prescription tranquilizer, Valium, "ranked second only to alcohol in combination with other drugs in abuse episodes treated in emergency rooms."

Drug interactions involving the minor tranquilizers can be dangerous or even deadly. When you're taking tranquilizers, it's best to avoid alcohol and get your physician's and pharmacist's guidance as to whether any other prescription or nonprescription medication you might need is safe to take at the same time.

You should also be aware that tranquilizers may lessen your alertness, which could make a crucial safety difference if you need to drive or operate machinery. Check with your physician about this too.

Tranquilizers aren't the only alternative to anxiety. Relief from tension should come by other ways and means. The "three R's of relaxation" can help us cope for a lifetime, may be cost free and can have some rather pleasant side effects.

Learn to recognize the warning signs of spiraling stress. How upset do you get when you lose your last dime in the phone booth, or the car behind you honks at you in traffic, or the waitress burns your toast? A pattern of big upsets over little things may mean you're living close to your boiling point.

Your body is also a revealing stress barometer. Mental tension is often reflected in muscle tension. One example is your jaw, says Jane Madders, MCSP, author of *Stress and Relaxation* (Arco Publishing Company). Do you unconsciously tense your jaw and clench your teeth tightly together? A continual habit of this can contribute to dental disorders and tension headaches, it's noted.

In general, experts say we should learn to listen to our bodies. They have characteristic ways of telling each of us when stress is reaching overload proportions: headaches, backaches, stomach problems, eating too much or too little, smoking or drinking more than usual, etc. Everyone's different. Learn the tension tip-offs that apply to you.

Something else you can do is reduce stress. Major changes in our life-style can be stressful, even when they're pleasant. Researchers Holmes and Rahe compiled a list of significant life changes which were assigned different point values. A high overall score correlated with a higher chance of having a major illness within two years. So it might be wise to *limit* life-style changes. If you've gone through a divorce or death of a spouse, for example, you might want to wait a while before you move your home or change your job.

Let go with laughter. Entertainer Bob Hope has called laughter an "instant vacation." Look for something humorous in a tense situation. Share a joke with others. Recall a funny episode from a similar incident.

A psychologist has said we can often bear stress better if at least one other person knows what we're going through. But if we come home at night "uptight" and "dump" on loved ones, the resulting row may *add* to stress. If this is your plight, it might help to set aside a brief "quiet time" when you first walk in the door so you can unwind alone in a way you find relaxing.

Finally, learn to release tension on a daily basis. Mental and muscle tension are interconnected. Relaxing either your muscles or mind can help the other unwind.

Put yourself in a *position* to relax. Any pose held long enough can tense your muscles, it's said. Muscles tighten, circulation lessens and you start feeling uncomfortable and achey. Movement contributes to relaxation, and can also boost mental alertness. A UCLA fitness expert found that of his students taking doctoral exams for four hours at a time, those who fidgeted kept up their performance better than those who sat still. He suggests it was due to a better blood supply to the brain.

If you sit quite a bit at work your chair may be very important. Make sure your chair is right for you. Madders advises, "It should give good but not exaggerated support for the lower curve of your back, your feet should easily reach the floor, the seat edge should not press on the soft structures at the back of your knee and the height should be such that you do not have to stoop or hunch your shoulders as you work." Another authority adds that ideally the chair should be comfortable in more than one position, to encourage movement.

Some form of regular, habitual physical activity suited to your health and conditioning level, interests and life-style can also contribute to relaxation. A simple one is walking more.

And how about a quick mental vacation for a few minutes a day? Find a spot where you won't be disturbed. Sit or lie down comfortably. Imagine yourself in a favorite place—such as lying on the beach. You can then focus on each area of the body in turn (left and right feet, calves, thighs, stomach, back, arms, neck, face) and feel yourself let go and relax each set of muscles in turn. End by lying quietly for a couple of minutes, count slowly backward, wriggle arms and legs a little and come back to the present.

You may be surprised what a big difference a little relaxation can make!

9

EXECUTIVE STRESS

by Dr. Arnold Fox and Barry Fox

If you're the average executive—you're overweight!

If you're the average executive—your cholesterol level is 230 plus!

If you're the average executive—you have a 1 in 3 chance of dying of a heart attack by age 60!

If you're the average executive—you couldn't walk the five or ten flights of stairs to your office!

If you're the average executive—stress is already taking its toll on your body!

If you're the average executive—you're scared! And you should be!

Do you know what the saddest part about all this is? Not enough people care—at least they don't seem to care; they don't do anything about it. Perhaps that's because it's now commonplace to spend the last 20 years of our lives under the constant care of a cardiologist: perhaps it's rather ordinary for someone you know to have had bypass surgery: perhaps we're not surprised anymore when a 45-year-old businessman drops dead of a heart attack: perhaps we figure we're all gonna get cancer sooner or later anyway.

The typical executive I see is in his forties. He's got a lot of money, a Mercedes, a swimming pool, an office on the twentieth floor in Century City. He also has chest pains, headaches which make it impossible for him to concentrate, he's tired most of the time, and he has no energy for a full life. He's put on a pound a year since age 25. He can't walk seven blocks without developing shortness of breath. Stress is taking its toll on this executive and he doesn't even know what stress is and how it affects him.

The average executive works too hard. He is too busy to enjoy life. He doesn't exercise; he eats "poison." Most damaging of all, he allows himself to be continually stressed. Stress is what is killing him. Of the 10 leading causes of death in this country today, eight are attributable to stress. Stress is the non-specific response of the body, mind, or emotions to any demand made upon them. Who makes the demand? *You do!* What kind of demand? *Any kind!*—from fighting with your spouse to eating a dough-nut. Any time you ask your body to respond to something, whether it be physical, emotional, or spiritual, you are stressing your body. An important point to remember is this: Stress is not what happens to you; it is how you take it. Being caught in traffic is not stress. *Getting mad* because you are stuck in traffic is stress. Working hard is not necessarily stressful. Working harder than *you* are able to is stress. While each stressor has its specific effects—some physical, some mental—all possess the common feature of requiring some sort of adaptation, some change, from your body.

The vast majority of the executives who come to see me can be helped very easily. If they follow the Anti-Stress Guide to the New Health (more about the New Health later), within four months they feel better. Their blood pressure is down, they have unlimited energy, their headaches and assorted pains are gone. They enjoy active lives.

They're out every morning jogging, walking briskly, or bicycling. Most important of all, they're happier than they've been in years.

Dealing with this type of patient is very rewarding, yet, at the same time, very frustrating. It's rewarding to help a person regain health and vigor without having to rely on pills and medications. In my 18 years of practicing traditional internal medicine and cardiology I was rarely able to restore a person to such vitality as I am able to now. On the other hand, it's frustrating because it is so hard to get through to people. People seem bent on destroying themselves, ruining their bodies and minds. Then they run to their doctor, hoping that by exchanging their money for his pills and surgery they will become healthy once again. Unfortunately, there isn't a pill that I, or any other doctor, can prescribe that will restore a person's vitality. Instead of ruining their health and throwing away their money chasing chimeras, people can enjoy a long, healthy, zestful, and happy life if they follow this simple, natural, fun prescription.

First, learn to look at health as a spectrum. Health is not an either-or proposition: either you're sick or you're not sick. Health ranges along a spectrum from what I call "The New Health," down to terminal illness and death.

At the top of the spectrum is "The New Health." The New Health is what we were all meant to have. The New Health is living young, healthy, strong, and happy to a very old age. The New Health is what Professor Hildebrand of UC Berkeley has: he's 97 years old, and five days a week he walks briskly up four flights of stairs to his office—without pause. His resting heart rate is 60 beats per minute—better than most 30-year-olds. Below "The New Health" is "Good Health." If you have Good Health you are functioning at near your highest potential. Next is "Fair Health." At Fair Health you don't feel all that good, but you don't feel bad, either. You have nothing wrong, but you haven't got much "get up and go." Next comes "Signs." These are the first measurable signs of illness. After "Signs" is "Symptoms." Symptoms are what the doctor can find. By the time you have symptoms of disease, you are far from optimal health. Most Americans fall between "Signs" and "Symptoms." Following "Symptoms" is "Measurable Illness." At this stage you have an identifiable, possibly serious illness. However, your health's degeneration is treatable and even reversible. Next comes "Chronic Illness," then "Death."

I tell my patients they could all have The New Health. The New Health is waking up in the morning after a good night's sleep feeling great, and ready to begin the day's work with a zest and a real joy of living. You should feel great, not just now but through your retirement years. You should feel wonderful without the use of alcohol, tobacco, stimulants, and anti-depressants. Your work should be meaningful and productive. Your love relationships should be profound and enjoyable.

Following is what I call "The Dr. Fox Anti-Stress Guide to 'The New Health.' " By following the simple rules in this guide you can live young to an old age.

Diet

Don't eat that doughnut—it will cause you stress!

What's this? Have doughnuts joined employers, traffic, and in-laws as stressors (substances which cause stress)? Absolutely! Stress is not only caused by such factors as love, hate, anticipation, anxiety, etc.; stress also results from eating certain foods which cause our bodily functions to be profoundly and adversely influenced. Stress is the non-specific response of the body, mind, or emotions to any demand made upon them. Eating certain food causes your body to focus its attention on that food because that food is in some way harmful. Your body is required to deal with that foodstuff, to control and dispose of it. That is stress.

When you eat a doughnut, the sugar in the doughnut causes your blood sugar to rise dramatically. Your body must respond to this rise in blood sugar by having the pancreas pump out insulin to drive the blood sugar down. This, in turn, causes the adrenal glands to attempt to stabilize the blood sugar by pouring out adrenal hormones.

That is stress! Eating a doughnut forces your body to respond to, and suffer through, drastic changes in blood sugar. Over the years your body will lose its ability to repair effectively and efficiently. Your body will begin to break down like an overused and abused machine.

How can you reduce stress? A very simple and positive step, one that will show almost immediate results, is to change your eating habits and adopt the Dr. Fox Anti-Stress Diet—the 13 commandments for healthful eating:

1. Your body is your greatest asset—honor it with healthy eating.

2. Stay as close to nature as possible in your eating. God made the food, and it's more likely the food is more healthy than if man made it.

3. Avoid food additives.

4. Take the proper amount of vitamins and minerals calculated for you.

5. Don't overeat.

6. Don't eat sugars.

7. Don't eat refined foods.

8. Don't eat salt.

9. Don't eat fats or oils.

10. Don't eat foods high in cholesterol.

11. Do eat complex carbohydrates.

12. Do eat plenty of fiber.

13. Do drink water (no coffee, tea, alcohol, soft drinks).

Remember, the body you have now is the only one you're going to have. Think of your body as a very complex factory. The raw materials brought to this factory are the foods and drinks you consume. From these raw materials are made the only thing you can't buy anywhere, for any price—your health.

This is how you should look at food and stress: Our bodies were designed to run on certain foods which contain all the necessary vitamins, minerals, proteins, etc. If you don't get enough of all the various nutrients, your body will not operate at full capacity. If you add to your diet food-stuffs which were not part of the original plan, you force your body to divert attention from the daily running of the body to dealing with the unwanted foodstuffs.

That is stress. Recall the discussion of doughnuts and stress. Yes, your body can deal with the stress caused by one doughnut, and maybe even the stress caused by one thousand doughnuts. But sooner or later your body is simply going to give up. Assaulted by demands to deal with doughnuts, sugars, fats, salt, additives, etc., your body will be overwhelmed. Your body will run panting from one harmful food to another, until it is no longer able to function the way it should.

The average American's diet is composed of the following:

- 40 to 45 percent of our calories come from fat.
- 40 percent of our calories come from carbohydrates. At least half of these carbohydrates are refined carbohydrates, such as white flour, cakes, etc. Refined carbohydrates are poison.
- 15 to 20 percent of our calories come from protein. (This is more than is necessary.)

The Dr. Fox Anti-Stress Diet, however, is composed of the following:

- 20 percent of the calories come from fat.
- 70 percent of the calories come from carbohydrates. (No refined carbohydrates.)
- 10 percent of the calories come from protein.

We should eat to live, not live to eat. We should eat only natural foods containing the necessary nutrients. We should not eat more than we need. We should not eat foods containing substances (fats, additives, sugars, salt, etc.) that cause our bodies stress.

Emotions and Stress

The average American is literally killing himself with stress. The way he lives, the way he reacts to ordinary and extraordinary events affects his stress level. Considerable research into stress-prone individuals indicates that there are three types of personalities—the A, B, and C personalities.

We all know the "Type A." He (or she) can be found in abundance in any office building. They're the hard-driving, excitable, volatile, success-oriented career person. Eyes glued to their watches, rushing from appointment to appointment, they're continually bombarded with stress. They allow no time to relax, to have fun. Their adrenals— the stress glands—pour lots of adrenalin into their veins. They're candidates for a heart attack.

On the other end of the spectrum is the "Type C" personality. These people tend to repress their feelings—turning their anger, impatience, and jealousy inward. This results in their adrenal gland being stimulated by the hypothalamus (the emotional control center in the brain) to produce cortisone-type hormones. Cortisone depresses the body's immune system, leaving the body open to attack from various ailments. "Type C" diseases include depression, arthritis, and cancer.

The "Type B" personality is the one we want to be. They're the ones who are able to handle the extremes of life. They take the time to relax after each stressful period. Some stress is unavoidable. "Bs" never allow the unavoidable, short-term stress to build into long-term stress and disease.

We can all learn to be "Bs." Here's what we must do:

1. Learn what stress is. Stress is not simply being yelled at by your boss. Stress is the non-specific response of your body to any demand made upon it. Your body does not get mad when you are caught in traffic. *You* get mad, and you force your body to respond to your anger. You are causing yourself stress! *Stress is not what happens to you; it's the way you accept what happens to you.*

2. We have to look at the pace of our lives. We must slow down, avoid too many changes. If you have the time to appreciate and become familiar with your surrounds, you are more likely to live healthy to an old age.

3. We must increase our resistance to stress so that when stress hits, we are better able to handle it. Follow the Anti-Stress Diet. The healthier your body is, the more resistant to stress it will be.

4. *Learn to relax!* The best way to deal with stress is to relax. If you're caught in traffic and you're late for an appointment, don't get excited. Getting excited will not get you there any faster. When you are unavoidably stressed, take 10 or 15 minutes to just sit down and relax, think about nice things. After work each day get rid of all the stress you are carrying around with you. When you come home you can meditate, jog, smell flowers, see a funny movie. Do anything you like, as long as it is enjoyable.

5. Decide what is and is not worth fighting for. If you're fighting for the big account, give it all you've got. *But remember*—not everything is worth fighting for. Assess each situation. Decide whether or not it's worth the stress.

Too many of us are becoming seriously ill in our forties; too many of us are dying in pain. Too many of us are dying old and broken and at a young age. We don't have to die at the too-young age of 60. We could all live young to a very old age.

6. I advise everyone to set up a health-care program. Don't rely on your doctor or other health-care professional to take care of you. *No one cares about you and your health as much as you yourself do.* Don't let your doctor get away with handing you some pills. Ask him exactly what is wrong with you. Make him tell you how you became ill. Use illness as an opportunity to learn more about your body.

Here at the American Institute of Health we make our patients learn about themselves. After a thorough examination, history, and tests, our patients all see our nutritionist. We demand of our patients that they learn how to eat right. The "Type A and C" personalities among our patients all see our behavior modification counselor, individually or in groups. I sit down with each patient and discuss my findings and recommendations. This discussion is taped; a copy is given to the patient. The patient is expected to listen to the tape and learn. You cannot delegate responsibility for your health to someone else. If you want to be healthy, if you want to have "The New Health," it's up to you.

THE HEALTH SPECTRUM →

THE NEW HEALTH

GOOD HEALTH

FAIR HEALTH

SIGNS

SYMPTOMS

MEASURABLE
ILLNESS

CHRONIC
ILLNESS

DEATH

10

HOW TO LOWER YOUR BLOOD PRESSURE

by Willa Vae Bowles

What Is Your Blood Pressure?

Your blood pressure is the degree of pressure exerted by your *heart* and *arteries* to keep the blood circulating in the tiny blood vessels through your body. Each time your heart beats the left ventricle of your heart propels the blood within it into a large artery called the *aorta*. From the aorta, the blood flows into many arterial branches which become smaller and smaller until they connect with the veins through the capillaries. Because of the FORCE with which the left side of your heart ejects the blood into the aorta, it flows with considerable speed, and a pulse wave is sent ahead through all the arteries. This pulsation is easily felt at the wrist. The arteries are elastic and flexible, and in the artery walls are muscle fibers which contract and help send the blood along. The combined effects of the force of pumping action of the left ventricle of your heart and the elastic contraction of the arteries serve to maintain a pressure within the entire arterial system. This is your blood pressure.

How to Measure Blood Pressure

Blood pressure is expressed by two figures such as 120/80. The maximum level is called *systolic pressure* which reflects the force exerted in the arteries with each heartbeat that propels the blood out of the left ventricle of the heart into the aorta. The minimum level is known as the *diastolic pressure* which records the least amount of pressure during the resting phase of the heartbeat. These blood pressure readings are taken to learn the force with which blood is pressing on artery walls.

The systolic and diastolic pressures are recorded by means of a *sphygmomanometer* (Greek term meaning measurement of pulses). There are many types of blood pressure instruments on the market today. I have an Electronic Self-Taking Blood Pressure Kit operated by battery so the readings are by flashing light and audible beep tone. It's a simple procedure, and you can easily learn to do it yourself.

Normal Range of Blood Pressure

Age	Male	Female
25-29	108-140/65-90	102-130/60-86
30-34	110-145/68-92	102-135/60-88
35-39	110-145/68-92	105-140/65-90
40-44	110-150/70-94	105-150/65-92
45-49	110-155/70-96	105-155/65-96
50-54	115-160/70-98	110-165/70-100
55-59	115-165/70-98	110-170/70-100
60-64	115-170/70-100	115-175/70-100
65 & older	115-175/70-95	120-192/65-102

There are wide variations in the so-called normal blood pressure at different ages. People vary in their response to everyday activities, change of posture, exercise and emotional stimulation. Blood pressure is not fixed nor does your blood pressure determine how you feel.

What Causes High Blood Pressure

It is agreed that high blood pressure appears between the ages of 30 and 35 and there is little likelihood of getting it after age 55. Many people have high blood pressure but do not know it. But despite the lack of symptoms, elevated blood pressure slowly and steadily damages your arteries, kidneys, heart and brain.

High blood pressure in itself is not a disease but is an effect caused by some disease process. The recording of high blood pressure is only the beginning of a health exam. Then the search begins to discover what part of the body is showing signs of inadequate blood circulation or a disease. Examination of the blood vessels in the retina of the eye often helps to determine the condition of the arteries in the rest of your body. If the problem is detected early, the damage can be reversed.

There are no symptoms that will pinpoint high blood pressure. It must be checked. However, some people have a persistent morning headache that diminishes during the day. Although there are sometimes complaints of inability to concentrate, insomnia, nosebleeds, numbness, or generalized weakness, some doctors feel it is the knowledge of having high blood pressure that produces a state of anxiety and tension which causes these symptoms.

When readings are repeatedly above 150/100, it indicates that the blood circulation is impaired. The amount of blood within the circulatory system, the thickness of the blood, and the amount of blood put out by the heart with each beat are other considerations. Unless corrective measures are taken, problems will soon develop. When the arteries that supply blood to the heart become hardened and narrowed, you can experience temporary heart pain, a serious heart attack, or an enlargement of the heart. When the arteries in the brain are hardened, a change in personality may be noticed, such as gradually becoming irritable and stubborn and experiencing lack of short-term memory. Or there may be a sudden stroke. When the kidney is damaged, you are apt to be weak and anemic and perhaps have swollen face and ankles.

If your recordings show consistent high blood pressure you need to have a complete examination to determine whether the heart, brain or kidneys have been affected. Carefully follow the doctor's or nutritionist's instructions to control the problem. In most cases, the exact cause of the high blood pressure cannot be isolated. Some things that may cause or aggravate the problem are:

1. *Heredity or environment.* You have followed the eating and daily routine habits of those you are around.

2. *Obesity.* Every pound of fat requires miles of extra blood vessels which place strain on your circulatory system.

3. *Salt.* Excess salt causes your body to retain fluid which in turn increases your blood volume.

4. *Stress.* Abnormal stress triggers the secretion of several hormones that raise blood pressure.

5. *Smoking.* Nicotine stimulates the adrenal glands which send out a hormone to help defend the body against this deadly toxin; the blood vessels constrict and the pressure goes up.

6. *High carbohydrate diet* can hinder the digestive system and function of the kidneys to properly filter the blood.

7. *Poor diet that has led to liver congestion.* Old poisonous waste from eating too much processed food, sugar, white flour, liquor, meats, etc., can clog the tissues of the liver.

8. *Tumors.* Occasionally a tumor on a gland or organ must be surgically removed and the person's blood pressure will return to normal.

9. *Endocrine glands*. Many women develop high blood pressure during menopause.

Low Blood Pressure

Approximately 25-30 percent of the population has low blood pressure, i.e., a recording of below 110/70. On the whole, these people lead normal, active lives with a greater-than-average life expectancy; however, some are underweight and narrow-chested and tire easily. Usually the lack of stamina is not due to the low blood pressure but rather to their circumstances and nervousness. The lowest blood pressure is found in patients with Addison's disease which can be corrected under the direction of a good doctor.

How to Control High Blood Pressure

1. *Drugs*. The doctor usually gives a supplement of potassium along with the medication. I suggest eating a banana and 2 tablespoons of hominy daily. *There can also be side effects to some drugs* such as nervous depression. Should this happen, contact the doctor immediately.

2. *Low salt diet*. Sometimes eliminating salt from the diet completely takes care of the problem. Even if a doctor prescribes a drug, he usually warns his patient to watch his salt intake. Whether you have high, low or normal blood pressure, it is wise to restrict your salt intake unless you are working out in the extremely hot weather. There are many flavorable seasonings on the market such as Vegit and Spike as well as good salt substitutes. Also cooking with herbs, spices, onions, garlic, peppers and kelp adds much interest to every meal.

3. *Avoid or greatly reduce* smoking and drinking of coffee, tea and alcohol.

4. *Reduce stress*. Even though we are often a victim of unplanned, stressful circumstances, our attitude toward

God and others is the key to keeping calm, relaxed and enjoying inner peace.

5. *Lose excess weight.* It is best to follow a well-balanced restricted diet tailor-made for you by a good doctor or nutritionist.

6. *Avoid white flour and sugar.* These add no vitamins or minerals to your body's upkeep; they are merely empty calories that hinder the absorption of the B vitamins and other nutrients. Cut out refined sugar from your diet and you'll cut down on stress.

7. *Exercise.* This cannot be overemphasized. Exercise daily by walking, swimming, tennis or anything you enjoy.

8. *Drink pure water.* Steam-distilled water is the purest, but be sure to take a multiple mineral supplement. Water is the catalyst in the human body, and you need plenty of it in order to help manufacture good blood and cells.

9. *Valuable lecithin* should be taken daily as it's beneficial for breaking up cholesterol and preventing the hardening of the inner lining of the arteries. Lecithin is the natural substance found in your trillions of cells and is necessary for the rebuilding of cells and for the metabolism of fats. Lecithin helps the oil-soluble vitamins A, D, and E to digest, which helps to build an immunity against viral infections.

10. *Miracle medicine food for high blood pressure: garlic.* Any nutrition book you read and many medical books will advise the use of *garlic* as the safest, most dependable food to relieve high blood pressure. No one can explain exactly why. But we cannot argue with success, especially when the only side effect is a garlic breath. And that can be tremendously helped by eating parsley, mint or orange peelings afterwards.

Garlic, raw or in tablet or capsule form, will not interfere with any other medication; however, you should discover that you can soon greatly reduce your medication. My mother, who was suffering from extremely high blood pressure, is now completely off all medication. But you should not go off medication until your doctor says so.

Garlic is helpful for many other disorders too. It is known as the poor man's antibiotic! It is very beneficial for the digestive system and aids in the elimination of toxins. It is a blood cleanser, stimulates blood circulation, normalizes intestinal flora, kills parasites, and helps to rid the body of excess phlegm and mucus.

Garlic should be used raw in cooking and salads. Food will soon taste flat without it! When traveling or eating out, take the tablet or capsule. You can purchase the tablets with parsley to help prevent body odors. While you are taking a large amount (garlic therapy, we call it), you may even notice the odor from the pores of your skin. Don't despair! The results are worth it. Soon you will be just on a maintenance amount of one tablet or capsule with each meal. But keep using the fresh garlic in food preparations!

11. *Vitamin Mineral Supplements*. It is best that you have a hair analysis in order to know the exact needs of your body. Most certainly you will want extra vitamin B complex, vitamin E to thin the blood and help with absorption of lecithin, and calcium to help calm the nerves. Your test may show you need some of the heavier minerals like zinc and selenium. Until you have your test results and recommendations by your doctor or nutritionist, I suggest you take a good high-potency multivitamin and chelated multimineral supplement. Also I suggest that daily you treat yourself to a cup of hot or cold watermelon seed tea or parsley tea. Another profitable habit is to eat asparagus three times a week to help break up oxalic acid crystals in the kidneys and strengthen the heart.

12. *Cleansing fasting*. Before any food-for-medicine therapy can be very effective, the body must be cleansed of

the accumulation of toxins. The seven-day detoxifying fast is excellent. Very busy people who do not take out time to rest and fast can eat lightly and take the product known as Sero-Detox distributed by Seroyal Brands. It is a formula of vitamin C and certain minerals.

Seven-Day Detoxifying Feast/Fast

If you are a diabetic victim or suffer with low-blood sugar (hypoglycemia) see your doctor before going on any fast.

Do not start unless you have dedicated intentions of staying on the feast/fast for the full seven days.

Be enthusiastic about your adventure. Form a mental picture of yourself with brighter, sparkling eyes, rosier cheeks, clear skin and much energy.

Do not plan to attend any banquets or eating celebrations unless you can arrange to have your needed foods. It is a matter of self-discipline. I have actually eaten at home and then attended a banquet for which I had paid a good sum, but I ate only the vegetable served and took the meat home to my dear dog. Other items I ignored.

Purchase at your grocery and health food store the things needed.

Recipe for Vegetable Broth

Place 2 quarts of distilled water in large vessel and bring to boil. Cut into small pieces 7 large carrots, a small bunch of celery, 2 medium-sized onions, 3 zucchini and add to the boiling water. Boil for 15 minutes. Add 1/2 bunch fresh parsley and 2 cups fresh spinach, cut fine. Boil another 10 to 15 minutes. Drain off the juice or broth. Vegetable or garlic salt may be added for flavor if desired. (If fresh spinach is unavailable, use a small box of frozen spinach. If zucchini is unavailable, use a few green beans . . . if neither is available, make the broth without them.)

This recipe makes a one-day supply. It can be used hot

or cold. The purpose of the broth is to flush. It is full of minerals.

You can put it in a thermos to take to your job.

Mornings: Squeeze the juice of 1 lemon into 8 ounces of hot water and drink 15 minutes before breakfast.

Breakfast: Orange or grapefruit juice (at least 8 ounces). Cottage cheese (5 level tablespoonfuls: no more or less). Fresh fruit (at least 1/2 pound of any fruit except bananas or avocados. Eat just one or a mixed fruit bowl). Herb tea (red clover, sage, parsley, chamomile, peppermint or any of your favorites).

Midmornings: You may have all the fruit juice or vegetable broth you want. Also eat fresh raw fruits.

Lunchtime: Vegetable broth (drink at least two cups during meal). Salad (make a vegetable salad from at least 4 of the following: artichokes, asparagus, beans, beets, brussel sprouts, cabbage, carrots, cauliflower, cucumbers, celery, dandelions, endive, eggplant, fresh green corn, fresh green peas, green peppers, kale, red-leaf lettuce, okra, onions, parsley, parsnips, radishes, rutabagas, spinach, swiss chard, tomatoes, turnips. Make a dressing of only olive oil, lemon juice and salt.

Afternoons. Between lunch and dinner drink all the vegetable broth or fresh vegetable juice you desire. Fill up; it is medicine for you. If you feel weary, eat some fresh fruit.

Dinner: Vegetable broth (drink at least two cups during meal). Steamed vegetables (select two or three from those listed above). Butter may be added for flavor. No potatoes. Baked apple with cream or a fresh fruit salad. Herb tea or water.

After Dinner: If you feel hungry before bedtime, drink more vegetable broth or fruit juice or eat fresh fruits.

Notes: The first day you may feel some slight discomfort. This is expected. There may be some headache, nausea, and gas pains. About the third or fourth day your bowels and kidneys will begin to move more freely. You may notice a thicker urine.

Globs of mucus may come up; if so, spit them out—do not swallow.

If you are constipated before beginning the feast/fast, take an Herblax the night before.

For the best results, I emphatically recommend an enema every night regardless of the number of movements during the day. The purpose of the enema is to remove from the folds of the colon and bowels any waste matter which may have remained lodged and which might otherwise be absorbed into the system during sleep. Use 2 quarts of water into which the strained juice of 2 lemons has been added. Or, you may use chamomile tea. Insert only about one cup of water at a time and massage the abdomen well so that it will go up the colon path; then add another cup.

Stay on this feast/fast diet for seven days and then gradually start adding whole-grain foods, eggs, cheese, lean meats into your diet again. You will never be sorry that you spent those seven days detoxifying your system. It will pay great dividends in better health.

Most authorities have concluded that when there are signs of high blood pressure, there is definitely a problem in the kidneys and/or liver. There are several methods of giving these organs a good cleansing. Methods I have proven helpful for the kidneys are:

Watermelon Fast. Cut watermelon in cubes and put one in your mouth every three minutes all day long. Eat or drink nothing else. Keep relaxed. You will be amazed at how much you can read in three minutes! Reset your timer, read, take another watermelon cube . . . for 8 to 10 hours. You will soon begin urinating more than ever in your life! Remember not to eat or drink anything else until the next morning.

Bartlett Pear Fast. If watermelon is unavailable, cut into cubes Bartlett pears and eat every three minutes. Fresh pears are best, but if unavailable, use sugarless canned.

Raw Beet Juice has been as successful as watermelon with some folk. Juice raw beets (if no juicer, put beets in blender with distilled water). Eat or drink nothing else all day—drink one teaspoon of beet juice every six minutes until you have consumed eight ounces of pure beet juice or 16 ounces if diluted with water. Your kidney tubes get the cleansing of their lives! You may pass some gravel or sulfa-formed crystals.

Wait at least a week, then cleanse your liver. Dr. Kelley's method has done wonders for many.

Kelley's Liver Cleanse. Make a punch in a gallon jar using the juice of 6 fresh lemons, 12 oranges and 6 grapefruit and fill to the top with distilled water.

Upon arising, take one tablespoon of Epsom salts dissolved in four ounces distilled water.

Repeat in 30 minutes. Repeat again in 30 minutes. (Total three doses.)

Two hours later begin drinking a glass of punch every one-half hour. In the evening you may have an orange or grapefruit. Keep relaxed while on this cleanse.

Liver and Gall Bladder Flush (wait a month after the Liver Cleanse). Monday through Saturday, *drink as much apple juice* as possible along with regular eating.

Three hours after good lunch on Saturday, take two tablespoons Epsom salts dissolved in one ounce of hot water. Follow with a little orange juice.

Repeat two hours later.

For dinner have a grapefruit or some grapefruit juice.

At bedtime, take one-half cup fresh lemon juice mixed with one-half cup warm olive oil. Go immediately to bed and lie on right side with right knee pulled close to chest for

30 minutes. Then you may sleep rest of night in desired position.

The next morning, one-half hour before breakfast, take two teaspoons Epsom salts dissolved in two ounces of distilled water.

Soon you should have some results with a bowel movement that will rid the body of much debris, perhaps green, irregularly-shaped objects varying in size from grape seeds to large grapes.

After your cleansing programs, keep on a good diet of much raw fruits and vegetables, whole-grain bread or cereal, moderate amount of protein from eggs, cheeses, fish, chicken and turkey, yogurt, and some lightly steamed vegetables. And eat plenty of GARLIC.

11

ANGER AND YOUR HEALTH

by Dr. Vernon J. Bittner

How you handle anger is important for your health. If you keep it inside it can cause depression, psychosomatic illnesses, and even lessen your immune system to fight such diseases as cancer. If it is expressed by putting others down, it can destroy relationships. But if it is handled constructively, it can be the energy to motivate you to change counterproductive behavior into productive behavior as well as be the tool for more intimate relationships.

Ephesians 4:25,26 states it this way: "Therefore, laying aside falsehood, speak truth, each one of you, with his neighbor, for we are members of one another. Be angry, and yet do not sin; do not let the sun go down on your anger."

Unfortunately, many do not see anger as a natural human emotion and that what makes it good or bad is how you handle it. Sometimes anger can do more good in society than love. Often anger toward injustices has led to more positive changes in our society than has a love for justice.

Many people seem to have a real problem with anger. Some people are not aware that they have it. Others do not connect anger with feelings like "upset," "frustrated," "disappointed" and "confused." Still others deny they are angry when they are in the midst of a rage. And even more use anger to cover up feelings like "fear" and "hurt," and are not aware that often anger is a secondary emotion.

The principles I am discussing in this chapter apply to you and me—we all have to know what to do about our anger.

Why Do We Try Not to Express Anger?

There are many reasons why people avoid expressing anger in a constructive manner.

"Nice people don't get angry at other people." This statement expresses both a misunderstanding of the Judeo-Christian religion and of good mental health. In the Old Testament God frequently demonstrated anger. If you read the Psalms you are aware that the psalmist is encouraged to express his anger to God so that he can get rid of it and be open to His will. Interestingly, there are many Psalms that begin with anger and end in the psalmist's being reconciled with God. This is also true of Christ in the New Testament—ie., even Christ was angry. I am not aware of any mental-health literature which indicates that having the feeling of anger is immature. Rather, one of the characteristics of a mature person is to be able to express anger constructively.

What people are really saying by "It isn't nice to get angry at other people" is: "I don't want to get angry and hurt others because they might hurt me back, and I don't want to get hurt." Most of us would feel more free to express our anger if we could be guaranteed that there would be no reprisal.

When we are angry at another person and express it, the recipient *may* feel hurt. If the anger is not expressed, it *can* hurt the person withholding it. The important issue is how it is expressed. To say, "I am angry at you because . . ." and tell the person why you are so angry is not as hurtful as telling the other off. The first way is simply an expression of how you feel, and the latter is putting the other person down. The difference is in the intention of the message. The first is intended only to convey a feeling and the second is intended to hurt. The New Testament has some good advice in this regard. We are told to "speak the truth in love."

"My anger will damage the relationship." If your friendship is that fragile you may not have one at all, because it is probably a rather superficial relationship. And if you lose it because you expressed how you felt, it probably was not worth having in the first place.

I have never seen a marital relationship destroyed by constructive anger, but many have been destroyed by anger expressed destructively. However, even more are destroyed because the anger is unexpressed. Soon the marriage dies because their repressed anger becomes a barrier to express love and receive it.

One of the positive things about expressing your anger constructively is that you will be able to know who your real friends are. They will not only be able to accept your anger, but will be willing to risk expressing their anger with you. This will also be a deterrent to attracting people who might like you only to use you or your friendship. "Con artists" do not spend much time with people who let them know how they feel about being had.

"Expressing my anger won't change things anyway." The primary reason for expressing your constructive anger is to help yourself, *not* the other person. Unless you truly believe it will help you, you probably will not do it anyway. The secondary reason is to inform the other person that you are angry and what angers you so that he is aware of the situation. This will help him to know what he can change to make the relationship better. Whether he chooses to change is up to him, but whether he does or not, you have still ben-

efited by expressing how you feel.

Telling someone else your angry feelings is also a sign of being a responsible person. First, it is taking responsibility for your own feeling of anger and being willing to handle it constructively. Second, it is being responsible *to* the other person to help that person grow. One of the most important ingredients in maturity is awareness—and self-awareness is gained primarily by how we are "mirrored" by others. It is impossible for you to stand outside yourself and see yourself as you are; therefore it is necessary for others to help you with this. Unless they are willing to be honest with you and be responsible *to* you and not *for* you, you will not grow in self-awareness and the process of maturity.

What Happens to Unexpressed Anger?

There is no such thing as unexpressed anger. Anger comes out one way or another. It is always expressed. The major concern is whether it is expressed constructively or not. When anger is not handled constructively, it does not go away. This is why it is so important to learn to handle it positively and why in the New Testament Paul says: "Do not let the sun go down on your anger." He, too, was aware that unresolved anger is destructive as well as sinful, because it has a negative effect on our health and separates us from others. Here are some expressions of anger:

"Gunnysacking." There are a lot of people who store up their anger and then when some unsuspecting person presses the right button they give them the whole load. Or they may express it in other destructive ways, like going on a binge, having an affair, quitting a job, having an automobile accident, or assaulting their spouses or their children.

The unfortunate thing about this behavior is that the "gunnysacker" feels justified in this kind of behavior. First, he has been "nice" for *so* long and has a right to be mean. Second, he has learned that this behavior is okay because it has been tolerated in the past and has gotten some results, even though it is counterproductive to him/her.

However, this method is quite destructive because the person who is on the receiving end of this anger is usually not aware of which behavior has resulted in the angry person becoming upset. Therefore it is impossible to change that of which you are unaware and so the relationship remains blocked. Besides, the reaction of the angry person is so inappropriate for the situation that the only results are confusion and alienation. If you are willing to learn to express anger as you experience it, you will eliminate having to gunnysack it and will increase the chances for expressing it positively.

Passive-aggressive behavior. Often repressed anger comes out in nondirective ways, consciously or unconsciously. It might be triggered by the person who motivated the anger or by some other cause. Also, by not expressing it directly but in a sly way, the angry person does not have to admit the anger or take responsibility for it. Passive-aggressive behavior is a learned life-style which can be changed if the person is willing to look at the fact that his behavior is motivated by anger.

There are various kinds of passive-aggressive behavior, such as *forgetting*. It is true that we all forget things at times, but there are some people who have difficulty remembering things. They forget what they do not want to remember, and most forgetting is intentional, either consciously or unconsciously. It is very frustrating to have a person on whom we depend to do something forget what he/she agreed to do. Many people hardly ever forget and others make a habit of forgetting.

Another expression of passive-aggressive behavior is *sarcasm*. This is "a nice way to be angry." Or another way of saying it is to tell someone you are angry at him/her with a smile on your face. It is giving a person two messages at once—both a compliment and a put-down. Like: "You look so nice I didn't recognize you." Or, "Your hair is awfully short, but I love it."

There are people who make these kinds of statements every day and wonder why people don't seem to want to be around them. After all, they are just having fun with them. Unfortunately, it is at the expense of the other person's being put down.

There are other ways that people are passive-aggressive too, such as *being late*. Many people come late to events unconsciously; this is their way of expressing their anger for having to be there.

I often experience this with people scheduled to see me. Maybe they are here because their wife/husband or parent asked them to come. They resent being asked and this is their vehicle for expressing their anger.

Unfortunately, most passive-aggressive behavior is unconscious and this is what makes it so difficult to change. You can't change something when there is no awareness of it. Unless someone lets you know how aggravating this behavior is, you will probably see no reason to change it.

Depression. Depression is one of the most common emotional problems in our culture, yet there are no statistics to verify this. The primary cause of depression is anger turned in at oneself or anger "bottled up." The individual who gets depressed (and we all get depressed at times) usually does not tell people how he feels, especially his feeling of anger. He has learned that it is all right to be angry at life or oneself but not at anyone else.

An example of this is the woman who is depressed and shows her anger at her husband by not taking care of the home or children.

One depressed wife told me, "I hate to be this way, but he will have to help me around the house for a change." The "for a change" was an indication of the anger she was feeling about her husband's neglect of her and the home.

In passing it should be noted, however, that there are other concomitant reasons for depression, like physical illness, fatigue, postpartum blues, and menopause in both women and men, to mention a few. But the primary cause is "bottled up" anger.

Psychosomatic disorders. There are physical problems caused by the failure to cope adequately with stress. The feelings that create stress are hurt, anger, guilt and fear. Anger, however, is a main cause of psychosomatic complaints, such as tension headaches, stiff necks, high blood pressure, lower-back pain, obesity, impotence and frigidity, ulcers, colitis, chronic itching, and even rheumatoid arthritis.

Besides anger-causing psychosomatic disorders, there is also evidence to indicate that people who fail to handle their stress properly are more likely to have cancer. The reason for this is that unresolved anger (stress) tends to affect a person's immune system so that he/she has less ability to fight disease—even the disease of cancer.

We as individuals have two options. We can deny our anger and keep it inside and thereby handle it in ways that are destructive to us and to others, or we can work at being more aware of it and express it directly and constructively, which will create a growing experience for ourselves and others.

These are some of the reasons why anger is not expressed and what happens to unexpressed anger that results in destructive behavior to oneself and others.

How Can I Handle Anger Constructively?

There are at least six steps involved in the process of expressing and resolving anger in a constructive manner.

Awareness. We have already discussed how deceptive anger can be and that we camouflage it in many ways.

Being aware of our anger is one of the most important ways of handling it in a healthy way.

There are many reasons why people have difficulty with this, and one of the most prevalent is the idea that healthy people are not angry. This is false. Healthy people *are* angry at times, but they have learned to express it constructively. Conversely, emotionally disturbed people do not have "too much" anger, but express it destructively. What causes a person to be healthy or unhealthy, not only emotionally but often physically and spiritually as well, is what he/she does with those feelings.

Therefore, the first thing we need in order to communicate anger constructively is an awareness of and a willingness to admit to our anger.

Identify the object. In order to deal with anger positively we must become aware of the person who is the focus of the anger. I may think that I am angry at my wife, but maybe I was angry when I walked into the house and my wife had nothing to do with what I felt. If I take the time to reflect on this, I will realize that I am angry at my boss.

The mistake many of us make is to take our anger out on the wrong person. Unfortunately, sometimes we act out the words in the old song: "You Always Hurt the One You Love." Sometimes we do that because we find it less threatening to be angry at our wife/husband than to express it to the appropriate person.

Have pure motives. This is hard to do because most of us have mixed motives most of the time for most of the things we do. We are human. We need to examine our reason for communicating our anger. Is it to help or hurt? If our primary purpose is to get back at the person rather than to remove the block to our communication (anger), we will end up losing.

Anger is a feeling to share, not a weapon to use to put someone down. It is a feeling that we may have because we care enough to get angry. But it is a feeling that must be expressed constructively; otherwise we will do more to destroy relationships than to restore them.

Don't bring up the past. The only issue that is relevant is the immediate one. There are, of course, exceptions to this, but don't "muddy" the discussion by bringing up the past. The only reason it is brought up most of the time anyway is to prove that you are right and the other person is wrong, and when this is done both lose.

Often when things finally do come out, it is because that person has been storing it for a long time and this was the "final straw." Then the anger is inappropriate for the situation, because the issue doesn't merit that much anger. I often tell people that if they fail to deal with past anger, they have no right to bring it up as part of their present anger.

Past angers only confuse the issue and make it difficult to sort out what is going on in the present. If we deal only with the current issue we have a much better chance of dealing with it in a reasonable way.

Discuss the real issue. Sometimes there is a primary issue and a secondary issue. The secondary issue is often the decoy because we are embarrassed to admit to ourselves and/or to others the real source of the anger.

The problem with a lot of us is that we don't always say what we mean. This often results in misunderstandings, hard feelings, and people isolating themselves from each other.

Express anger positively. A person can be very hurt and angry and still express anger in a constructive way. A constructive framework for expressing anger is: "Because I care about our relationship I want to share how I feel."

In Ephesians 4:15, we are encouraged to speak the truth in love. If we avoid saying what we mean we avoid relationships, and when we express it to hurt we sever relationships. Either way we lose. We need to express our anger in a loving way—because we care about the other person.

There should be no name-calling, accusations or unfair fighting. Calling others names is only to put them down. Accusing others is not being willing to look at your part of the problem. And fighting unfairly will only allow you to win the battle but lose the war. They are all counterproductive ways of expressing anger.

Communicating anger constructively means that we say what we mean and even quarrel without putting the other person down. We need to remember that our relationship is important, we are both worthwhile people, and we need to resolve our anger in a positive way.

Communication takes practice and so does expressing our anger if it is to be done in a healthy manner. Hopefully, anger can be seen as something that doesn't have to be feared, but as an opportunity for growth.

How Do You Prevent Anger?

There are some who would say there is no such thing as preventing anger. After all, anger is a feeling and feelings are neither right nor wrong; *they just are*. This is true; yet I am free to choose to be whatever person I want to be. This includes choosing feelings. I can choose to feel kindness or I can choose to feel anger by hanging on to how another person has hurt me. By saying this I am not saying that anger is an inappropriate feeling. At times anger is a justifiable emotion but not to the degree that you exclude other feelings, wallow in it, or use it to cover up feelings such as hurt. The anger discussed in this article will be the anger that is not only inappropriate but useless as well, and needs to be prevented.

One of the most important ways of preventing useless anger is to recognize that anger may be the result of feeling hurt. The difficulty with many of us is that we do not *act* on our feelings; rather we *react* to our feelings. The reaction to hurt is anger. Acting on the feeling of hurt would mean to express our hurt feelings in a constructive way, like: "I am really hurt when you don't come home from work because it seems that your buddies are more important to you than I am."

If you are willing to make a statement like the one above you will do several things. First, you will tell the other person exactly how *you* feel. Second, you will not cover up how you feel. Third, you will be stating why you have the feeling. Finally, you will be letting the person know when that behavior results in your feeling hurt.

Not only is it important to recognize that anger may be the result of hurt, *but feeling angry may also be the result of fear.* Anger is often a secondary emotion (reaction) to both hurt and fear.

Have you ever noticed that one of the times you seem to be the most aggressive is when you are the most afraid or feeling insecure? We all "whistle in the dark" at times. This is not all bad except when it involves relationships. Then it is a form of covering up our feelings and it becomes destructive to relationships because it is game playing.

As stated above, anger is sometimes the reaction to fear and insecurity. *If you carry this theory farther it would seem important to work on one's self-worth.* Feeling good about oneself could eliminate some of the anger you have. A definition I have used for anger is: "What causes anger is what someone says or does that threatens my self-worth as a person"—and if I do not like myself as much as I should I will be easily threatened.

There are many theories proposed for working on one's self-worth, but the most productive one is changing destructive behavior. For example, you cannot like yourself *if you do not like what you do.* If you have a volatile temper, this will reinforce the negative thoughts you have about yourself. Therefore, changing your behavior requires making a conscious effort to handle your anger appropriately. This may mean walking away temporarily to cool off, not storing up your anger, expressing your anger in the situation when you feel it, putting your anger in the form of a statement as discussed above, finding another person with whom you can discuss your feelings, and discovering other ways of working it out, such as exercise. You have to like what you do to like yourself, and the more you like yourself the more you will be able to prevent the occurrence of inappropriate anger.

The fourth method of preventing anger is: *Do not have expectations of people who have not earned your respect.* There are many people you can respect because they have been faithful in their relationships with you. There are others who are inconsistent and in whom you would be naive to put your trust. And there are many more you do not know at all. The difficulty you may have, however, is forgetting that there are some who will not fulfill the expectations you have of them. This is especially true if that person is important to you—like a spouse, a colleague, or a boss. Many times our *anger is nothing more than unfulfilled expectations*—and they are expectations you should not have had.

Another reason why anger becomes the feeling of choice is because of the frustration involved in trying to control or change other people. The only person you can change or control in any way is yourself. No matter how hard you try to control the behavior of another person, you will be unsuccessful unless he/she wants that as well. *You need to accept that you cannot control or change anyone else.* Otherwise you will have difficulty preventing useless anger from occurring.

Finally, you will not be able to do much to prevent useless anger if you do not have a forgiving attitude. *You must forgive the past!* If you hang on to the past hurt and anger, it will not take very much for someone to push the right button because *you are already angry.*

Forgiving the past does not mean that you like what has happened, nor that you believe it changes (because it may never change); it means simply that you let go of it so *you can feel better.* However, forgiving is not an easy task. Unless you want to forgive more than you want to stay angry it will not happen. As stated earlier, anger is a choice. Forgiveness is a choice, too.

These are some of the ways that you and I can avoid useless and inappropriate anger. You need to remember: Stress created by anger can be constructively handled and even prevented at times, because feelings *are a choice.*

I hope that you see that anger can be constructively communicated and that fighting can occur without one person attempting to damage the other. The difficulty in putting these principles into action is halfway between how simple it looks on paper and how impossible it looks in the midst of intense anger. Like anything else, it takes practice. If you will work at it in a methodical way initially, it will become a more spontaneous expression of living. When one gets to this point, anger is no longer frightening, but an opportunity for growth and maturity.

12

WHAT IS PEACE OF MIND?

by Dr. Vernon J. Bittner

I

In a recent Louis Harris survey people were asked to check which one or two items were the most important for their lives. "Good health" was at the top of the list, but second-most important was "peace of mind."

As a marriage and family therapist this seems to me to be one of the primary concerns of people who come to see me. In fact, most people feel that life is either empty or overwhelming. This is why they come. They are hoping to find something that will give a purpose to and direction for their lives.

Admit to being human. This is the first step toward finding peace of mind. Unless a person is willing to admit to being out of control in at least one area of life, either in the present or the future, there is no hope for finding serenity. This is true not only for the person who seeks counseling but also for those who don't. Everyone has limitations. No one is perfect. All people have at least one area in which life seems to be unmanageable. No matter how competent a person is, there is always room for growth. Initially, peace of mind means that one must admit to one's humanness.

Seek help from a higher power. To accept that we are human carries with it the idea that we need a power greater than ourselves to help us; for me, this power is God. But in order to make use of this power we have to be willing to turn our life over to His care—as we understand Him.

Finding this power and putting it to work in your life involves an act of the will. You have to be willing to risk. Unless there is a solution for the things that we cannot control, there can never be any peace of mind.

Turning our lives over is difficult. God is forgiving and accepts us as we are. Unfortunately, at one time in my life I did not see God that way. He seemed to be punitive, legalistic and unaccepting. Eventually I began to see His love. But still I found it hard to let go.

Being willing to trust is scary even when you're a secure person. If you are honest with yourself you know you are not in charge of your life all of the time, and yet you're expected to give the part that you *are* managing to a higher power. This seems to contradict all logic. However, the opposite is true. We are only able to find this power for our own lives, and be the persons we were created to be, and have meaning for our lives. This begins when we make the choice to rely on a power greater than ourselves. Trying to find peace of mind by yourself will not work.

There are some who might see this as a neurotic dependency and a sign of irresponsibility. Instead, He brings you strength to take responsibility for changing what you can change instead of wanting others to do it for you.

Perhaps the most threatening part of turning our lives over is not knowing in what direction it will take us. Yet the ultimate peace which all of us seek can only be found outside ourselves.

There are those who would sacrifice anything to gain power, to be successful and prestigious in the eyes of the world, or to avoid facing the consequences for inappropriate behavior. This will not give us the serenity that will last; it is only a way some people live in order to experience the temporary joys of life. These are most often a substitute for the real thing.

Many of us want God like we want an electric blanket—a little temporary comfort on a cold night, but then to be pushed away when the warmth of morning comes. God is not like a magic genie who can be summoned to turn our garbage into gold and our slums into palaces. Nor must we bargain with Him as Jacob did: "If God will be with me and will keep me on this journey that I take, and will give me food to eat and garments to wear, and I return to my father's house in safety, then the Lord will be my God" (Gen. 28:20,21).

Know your strengths and weaknesses. Making a realistic assessment of yourself is a difficult and sometimes painful process. Most of us are good at analyzing another person and prescribing what is necessary for their happiness, but when it comes to ourselves, we are either blind or cowardly.

A personality trait can either be an asset or a liability—it can either bring calmness to our lives or it can cause us physical, emotional or spiritual pain. For example, I used to take pride in my ability to be forgiving and understanding. Unfortunately, that also had its negative side because there were times when I would be so forgiving and understanding that I let people walk on me. Here a "good" trait, carried out to an extreme, became a character defect because I put myself through unnecessary pain. If this pain was not dealt with constructively and if I did not change the destructive behavior, I would continue to set myself up for further hurt.

Becoming aware of ourselves can be a very distressing process. We might find it to be a fearful or depressing experience—as well as one that could liberate us. This is not a one-time task, however; it must be a way of life.

To help you gain awareness of yourself, I would like to

suggest you use the following character traits as a basis for evaluation. This is a list of personal liabilities and assets used by persons for self-knowledge. This will help you to identify them and start you on your way to a more serene life-style. Reflecting on your strengths and weaknesses could best be done in solitude.

ASSET	LIABILITY
Faith	Fear
Self-respect	Self-pity
Love	Resentment
Understanding	Selfishness
Forgiveness	Guilt
Responsibility	Phoniness
Honesty	Dishonesty
Humility	False pride
Thankfulness	Hypercriticism
Patience	Impatience
Promptness	Procrastination
Reason	Rationalization

As you study this list, ask God to show you how some of your character traits become liabilities instead of assets.

● Do not rationalize.

● Admit the real reason for your difficulty no matter how distasteful it may be.

● Do not attempt to justify inappropriate or destructive behavior.

● Do not confuse bad temper with righteous indignation.

● Do not confuse stubbornness with determination.

● Do not allow your selfish pride to become "the right" to which you are entitled.

● Do not justify your faulty relationships with others by thinking that you have a right to your own opinion.

● Be open to the Spirit of God.

When we face ourselves, we discover our strengths and weaknesses, fulfill our human potential, and work toward experiencing a life of power, joy, serenity and love.

Share your problem, defect or sin. When we have become more fully aware of who we are, it is important not to live alone with our problems, defects or sins. These unspoken concerns could trouble us and even inhibit us from finding peace of mind. Unexpressed personal conflicts can grow like a cancer. They must be removed. This can be as painful as surgery. Sometimes it is not enough to admit the things that bother us; it is also necessary to talk to another trusted person. Unfortunately, many of us would rather suffer alone in silence than to confess our sins to someone else.

The practice of confessing our faults to another person is an ancient one. It was common in biblical times and it has continued to the present. It is not only a valuable principle in religious life but is now encouraged by psychiatrists, physicians, psychologists, social workers and other health-care professionals. It is also the basis of most self-help groups like Alcoholics Anonymous, Overeaters Anonymous, Gamblers Anonymous and other 12-step programs.

Unresolved guilt can be one of the most powerful forces in life. It can motivate us to change that which is destructive in our lives, or it can prevent us from being what God created us to be. Guilt is constructive in our lives only when we use it to change that which we do not like about ourselves.

There are two kinds of guilt: real and neurotic. We feel real guilt when we go against our moral value system. This guilt has a rational basis. Neurotic guilt is feeling guilty when we shouldn't. It is irrational. Children sometimes feel responsible for their parents' divorce, or feel that they fall short of the expectations of their parents. Hence they feel false or neurotic guilt. People who seem to feel guilty and apologetic about almost everything they do probably are suffering from neurotic guilt.

There are some persons in our society who feel that guilt has no value at all. This is hard to understand because there are times when we should all feel guilty. People who never experience guilt are either psychopathically ill or have ceased to be human. They lack a conscience and will probably end up outside the law; or they may abuse others to satisfy their own needs.

Repressing feelings of guilt can become a destructive force in our lives. The only way to resolve guilt is to be experiencing a sense of forgiveness. However, making God's forgiveness our own is sometimes difficult. Often we need to make confession to another trusted person. We need to be forgiven as we see in Matthew 18:18,19: "Truly I say to you, whatever you shall bind on earth shall have been bound in heaven; and whatever you loose on earth shall have been loosed in heaven. . . . If two of you agree on earth about anything that they may ask, it shall be done for them by My Father who is in heaven."

Confessing the things that bother us to someone else whom we trust helps to break with the past so we can begin a more constructive life-style. In addition, sharing what we are troubled about with another person usually helps us see that it is not as overwhelming as we thought. Also, experiencing the acceptance of another human being, in spite of the fact that he/she knows all about us, helps us to experience God's acceptance. Confession can help us understand why we did what we did, so we can avoid doing it again.

Finally, *unless we admit to being sinners, we will never admit to needing God, and we will not move toward finding peace of mind*. Almost every day I see people who are anxious, angry and discontented about life. This usually is a result of unresolved guilt and pain of the past. There is only one solution to this problem and that is to let go of the past. To admit it to ourselves, to believe that there is a power greater than ourselves who can transform us, and to confirm that we have God's forgiveness through the acceptance of others are the steps toward finding peace of mind.

II

In my work as a marriage and family therapist, the most common complaint of hurting people is that they feel unloved. Feeling loved is vitally important in finding serenity. So often I see people whose behavior can be summed up by a person walking around shouting: "Lord, please let someone love me."

People go through all kinds of things in an effort to manipulate someone to love them. And that is the basis of most personal and family problems.

On the other hand, healthy people who are in meaningful relationships with people and God are looking for people to love. These people have discovered that they are loved when they are willing to risk loving others. It is a hard lesson to learn, but life is much improved when we learn it. However, there are certain steps necessary to experience the peace of mind that loving and being loved can give.

First, we must be willing to remove the destructive aspects of our lives. Letting go of destructive character traits in ourselves is a very difficult process. There seems to be an unholy comfort in hanging on to the destructive patterns in our lives because they are familiar and predictable. Also, we didn't get them overnight and so it will take time to overcome them.

Many people, for example, have not learned to express anger, and so they bottle it up. This practice eventually creates depression, causing the angry person to withdraw from relationships, or it forces him to explode his stored-up anger inappropriately. This does not produce serenity. Yet it is difficult for a person to change his behavior because usually it occurs automatically. Unfortunately, the person who is depressed or who explodes for no apparent reason is hard to love.

Second, we must make a conscious effort to change our destructive life-style. When we have become aware of our defects and we want to have God help us to remove them, we have to commit ourselves to the task. It is not enough to *try.* "Trying is lying!" The only way change will occur is if we are committed to change.

The reason change is difficult is because some people are afraid to give up destructive attitudes like anger or fear. For some, these feelings have been with them so long they seem almost like friends. For example, anger for some serves as a defensive shield against being hurt—and at the same time it prevents them from experiencing love. Fear also serves some people well, because it becomes their excuse for avoiding what they do not want to do—and prevents them from experiencing meaningful relationships.

In addition, some people resist change because they would like to think they are controlled by a power outside of themselves. Usually this is an unconscious way of avoiding responsibility for one's own life.

Perhaps, though, the most obstructive deterrent to finding serenity is being possessed by an attitude of false pride which prevents us from seeing that we need God's help to change. Unless we give up our false pride we will deceive ourselves into thinking that we do not need to rely on God. Unless we let go of it, we will not want Him to remove our shortcomings—from within and without—that get in the way of finding serenity.

God created us for life and not death, for fellowship and

not isolation, for health and not illness, and for serenity and not turmoil. He wants us to have peace of mind. When we have asked God to help us remove our shortcomings so we are in a better position to give and receive love, we are on our way to finding serenity.

Third, we need to be willing to make amends or be reconciled with those we have harmed by thought or deed. Not only is it difficult to like ourselves if we are alienated from some of the important people in our lives, but it is impossible to have a relationship with God. And if there is no relationship with God and we feel estranged from some significant people in our lives, there is no serenity.

To make a list of those we have harmed and to become willing to make amends is very difficult. If we have lied to them or cheated them we have probably caused them spiritual and emotional pain. If we have an uncontrolled temper, we may have hurt them physically and emotionally. If our sex life is selfish, we may have caused misery and a desire for retaliation. There are more subtle ways of harming others too, such as being irritable, cold, irresponsible, impatient, grumpy, or domineering. Or we may wallow in depression and self-pity.

Besides making a list of those we have harmed, being willing to make amends, and changing our behavior, we also need to restore broken relationships with people. If we have to apologize and make up for harmful behavior we are less likely to repeat it.

Many people want to have God on their side, but they do not want to give up a resentment or grievance. If only they will make a list of those they resent, seek them out if possible, talk things over, forgive them so they can get rid of the malice in their hearts, they will experience joy, peace and serenity.

In order to claim our forgiveness, we need to forgive those who have injured us or are in our debt. There is no other petition in the Lord's Prayer that has a condition attached to it except this one: Forgive us our debts, as we also have forgiven our debtors" (Matt. 6:12). The condition here is that unless I forgive I will not be forgiven.

Becoming aware of those we have hurt involves recalling the hostilities, fears, conflicts, sorrows, guilts, and painful memories of the past. Most people are controlled more by their unconscious thoughts than they are by their conscious thinking. It is estimated that 70 percent of our behavior is motivated by our unconscious mind. If this is true, then it is apparent that we need to become more aware of ourselves. Otherwise we will not be able to do anything to resolve those negative attitudes which result in no peace of mind.

Conscious knowledge of those feelings that we need to resolve is difficult enough, but when we are not aware of what we are feeling—let alone not having reconciled these feelings—we may need some help in identifying them. Here are some ways of becoming aware of unconscious thoughts:

1. Talk about your feelings with someone you trust.
2. Write down the feelings.
3. Record your dreams.
4. Reflect on your past destructive behavior.
5. Meditate and pray.

I regret that space does not allow me to elaborate on these points, but these are some of the methods that may help you to recognize those you have harmed by thought, word or deed. These are the people with whom you need to make amends. Becoming aware of these conscious and unconscious memories that need healing is necessary to maintain your peace of mind and your health.

Making direct amends wherever possible is a discomfort many of us would like to avoid. We need to start with the primary people in our lives, like spouses, parents, children, and siblings. "There are others that we have harmed who are not any less significant as far as obtaining our serenity, such as relatives, friends, neighbors, and other acquaintances. There will also be those that we will be unable to contact either because they are deceased, or because we do not know where they are. There will be others where efforts toward reconciliation are better left undone because it may result in more injury than healing.

"The key to making amends is not only to be willing, but to have a loving and forgiving attitude."[1] Unless we come in this frame of mine we will blow our chances for reconciliation and serenity.

When we make amends it is also important not to dupe ourselves into believing that time will heal. What a terrible con job we are doing on ourselves! Time will not heal a burst appendix nor will it heal a feeling of guilt or resentment. All of these need surgery—either physical or spiritual. Spiritual surgery requires the painful process of setting right our relationships with people. Neglect this surgery and the body may become sick and destroy itself physically, emotionally, or spiritually. This is not a threat but a reality.

I am reminded of the man who was suffering from bleeding ulcers. He was filled with unresolved resentment toward many people who had hurt him throughout his life—people who had taken advantage of him, partly because he had allowed them to do it. However, he was unable to accept his part of the problem and refused to let go of his anger. Finally surgery was required for his ulcer. He lost three-fourths of his stomach. Within a short time his ulcer returned and he was again finding blood in his stool. This unresolved resentment (and the ulcer) continued until he was found dead in his apartment. He had bled to death because he refused to resolve his anger by forgiving those people who had hurt him. He refused to make amends.

Another way we fool ourselves is to believe we can get

along without other people. Maybe there were times in life when we were hurt by others so we came to the conclusion that the way to avoid this is to steer clear of people. It is true that many people are unlovable, vain, cruel, selfish, critical, and unsympathetic. But withdrawing from them is not the way to escape our need to make amends.

Often we feel like avoiding those who resent us. After all, who likes to be around angry people? But maybe we need to hear what they have to say to us. This does not mean that we let them abuse us, but perhaps there is some truth behind their anger—otherwise they would not be angry. If we keep fleeing from people who might injure us, acting as though we are always the innocent ones, we may never discover how we might have wronged them. Jesus said: "Love your enemies, and pray for those who persecute you" (Matt. 5:44). This means that we are not to flee from them or resent them but forgive them, make amends, and be willing to listen to them. Maybe this is why religion is sometimes referred to as "soft" and why some agnostics see it as an infantile attitude toward life, because we flee from our enemies and use our religion to escape life instead of using it to face life and love our enemies.

I remember a pastor friend of mine who was having difficulty in his parish. The people had taken one minute incident, removed it from its context, and blown it out of proportion. They wanted to get rid of their pastor because of his confrontive ways of dealing with people; but this had been concealed in the other accusation.

My friend had worked hard with these people and together they had accomplished much in the church. To have it all end this way was more than he could take. He began to isolate himself from his enemies in the congregation. One day he went out for a long walk in a wooded area near his home, which he had often done to get away by himself. As he left the road to enter the woods he heard the sound of footsteps behind him. He looked behind him but could not see anyone. He thought walking in the woods would allow him to be alone with God. He began to pray. Then he heard the footsteps again. He became so disturbed and frightened that he began to run along the path. He stopped two or three times to listen and each time he heard the noise of people walking behind him. He felt like a man pursued. He felt frantic and desperate. He recalled wanting so much to get away from people and to find a refuge in God. But he continued to hear the feet. Finally he decided to sit down and face who or whatever it was. But no one came; the sound of the feet disappeared and he heard God's voice within telling him that the feet were his and that the life that excludes people cannot find God either.

Please do not misunderstand me. There are times when we must avoid certain people. We need to take time to be alone and it becomes necessary to shut out the demands of people and things. At times it is appropriate to use God as a refuge, a hiding place, a retreat, but then we need to go back to people and to our enemies, forgiving them in spite of their criticism, loving them in spite of their disapproval, but not needing to like their meanness, to trust their disloyalties, or to believe that they will make amends with us. Through this experience we can be strengthened.

There are also times when we need to avoid other people because of their unwillingness to be reconciled with us. There is no benefit in allowing others to abuse us. This only enables them to be irresponsible and results in our martyrdom. Continuing to try to mend relationships with some people can be a waste of time and energy. And if we persist in setting ourselves up for hurt and rejection, we may need to examine why we do it. Perhaps it is because we think we need the forgiveness of these people in order to forgive ourselves. We don't! The only forgiveness we need is God's.

Making amends with specific people is one of the most

important aspects in finding peace of mind.

The fourth element that is important in experiencing serenity is to reflect daily on our behavior and when wrong to promptly admit it.

Taking a personal inventory every day includes not only what we did wrong but what we did that was right. Otherwise we will never be able to work toward fulfilling our potential as a person. Here we are to be aware daily of our strengths and weaknesses related primarily to our relationships. We find serenity by being committed. We find our lives not by holding on to them, not by jealously guarding them, but by freely giving them and by losing them in caring for others. As Jesus said, "Whoever wishes to save his life shall lose it; but whoever loses his life for My sake shall find it" (Matt. 16:25).

Finding peace of mind requires the same thing. It will never happen by spending all of our time looking within. We need to look at our relationships and work at correcting what went wrong so serenity can be ours.

Another vital part of the process toward finding peace of mind is having the added dimension of a meaningful meditation and prayer life. This is especially important when we experience the pain and brokenness of the world. Eventually this catches up to all of us. All too soon we experience hurt, fear, alienation, loneliness, and tension. Inevitably our bodies age, our dreams crumble, and our loved ones are lost. Unless we have the sense of knowing that we are not friendless, powerless, and hopeless, we will have a difficult time knowing any serenity. Prayer and meditation can help us know that we do belong to God.

Finally, peace of mind can be ours if we are willing to share the joy we have found in loving and being loved by God and others. This is one of the most difficult things for many of us to do. Perhaps we are afraid that what we have found will be unacceptable. We must share it or we will lose it. Our serenity is affirmed through the process of sharing. Through sharing we continue to grow and mature as persons in the fullness of the joy and peace we have found. Unless we do this, we will not find the serenity to practice what we have learned when we have to face the difficulties of life.

May God help us to be committed to finding serenity, knowing that it involves being at peace with God, our neighbor, and ourselves—as well as sharing it with others.

Notes
1. Some of the material that follows is from Vernon J. Bittner's *You Can Help with Your Healing* (Minneapolis: Augsburg Publishing House, 1979).

13

CARBOHYDRATES

by Dr. Eppie Hartsuiker

Energy is a much discussed subject these days. The supply of rich accessible fuels is rapidly being depleted by modern technology. But man is reluctant to accept the inevitable—that he must curtail his use of these rapidly depleting, comparatively expensive sources of fuel and be prepared to pay more for future energy.

The human organism also needs fuel for energy to carry on bodily functions. This it obtains from food sources. The growing populations of the world require cheaper and more accessible sources of energy, cheaper and more food. Energy for the body is supplied by three nutrients only— protein, fat and carbohydrate. (Alcoholic beverages also supply energy but are not considered a nutrient as such.) Minerals and vitamins do not provide fuel. Energy in foods is calculated as calories, more precisely as kilocalories, or sometimes called the big calorie. One gram of protein supplies four calories (kilocalories), one gram of fat nine calories, and one gram of carbohydrate four calories. Since fat provides twice the energy of protein or carbohydrate it would appear that it would be more economical to utilize more fat in the diet for bodily energy needs. However, fat is an expensive source of energy. For example, many ears of corn are needed to make one tablespoon of corn oil, whereas the same amount of corn-on-the-cob would provide a cheaper source of energy. Animal protein is also expensive. It requires many acres of grain to fatten cattle for market. Carbohydrate is the most inexpensive and abundant source of energy for the body.

The human diet includes grains, nuts, fruits and vegetation from the plant kingdom as well as meat, poultry and fish and other animal products used as food by a particular group of people.

The bulk of calories necessary for survival is derived from carbohydrates. Most societies depend upon a single type of grain or tuber as their main source of carbohydrate.

In human nutrition there is no definite requirement for carbohydrates. There does not appear to be a specific amount that must be ingested to be most healthful. The intake of foods rich in carbohydrate varies widely among individuals as well as in different parts of the world. This may be due to the availability and cost of protein-rich and fat-rich foods rather than a preference for cheaper carbohydrate-rich foods. Pound-for-pound, carbohydrate-rich foods are a much cheaper source of energy than protein or fat. There does not appear to be any health hazard from ingesting largely carbohydrate-rich foods, provided that they supply an adequate amount of minerals, vitamins, essential amino acids and essential fatty acids.

Carbohydrates are made up of elements of carbon, hydrogen and oxygen. The prefix *carbo-* stands for its carbon make-up. The proportion of hydrogen to oxygen is the same as found in water—two parts of hydrogen to one part of oxygen. Hence the suffix *-hydrate*, indicating this identical proportion of hydrogen and oxygen to water. Carbohydrates are sugars or complex compounds made up of many sugar groups, such as starch. The carbohydrates are classified into three categories as to the size of their molecules and their complexity. They are as follows:

1. The simple sugars. These are called *monosaccharides*, meaning that there is only one sugar group in each molecule.

2. The double sugars. These are called *disaccharides*, meaning that there are two sugar groups in each molecule.

3. The *polysaccharides*. These are large molecules consisting of many sugar groups.

The three most important simple sugars in the diet are *glucose, fructose* and *galactose*. The simple sugars really form the basis for all carbohydrates and all of these compounds that are found commonly in foods or in the body are sugars that contain six carbons or multiples of them. The most important double sugars are *sucrose, maltose* and *lactose*. In digestion these double sugars are broken down into the simple sugars. Hence, sucrose breaks down into glucose, and lactose into glucose and galactose. The polysaccharides include starch, dextrins, cellulose, hemicellulose and glycogen (animal starch). These more complex carbohydrates must be broken down into the simple sugar groups by digestion before they can be absorbed and used by the body.

All the carbohydrates from food are supplied by the plant kingdom with the exception of lactose, which is called milk sugar. Sugars are very soluble in water and they are easily transported from one part of the plant to another in the sap. The sugars are stored in the juices of fruits. The chief carbohydrates in fruits are the simple sugars glucose and fructose and the double sugar sucrose. Young fresh corn and green peas owe their sweet taste to the presence of sugar which is converted to starch as they mature, hence the practice of harvesting these crops when their sugar content is optimal and transporting them immediately to the processing plants to retain their optimal sweetness. Other vegetables that contain appreciable amounts of sugar are beets, carrots, onions, turnips, yellow winter squash and sweet potatoes or yams. The banana is starchy when immature. When it ripens the starch is converted to sugar.

Sucrose is the most popular double sugar and carbohydrate used on the table and in cooking. It is crystallized from juices extracted from the sugar beet or sugar cane. Another commonly used sugar is honey. It is approximately 50 percent glucose and 50 percent fructose. The higher proportion of fructose in honey makes it sweeter than sucrose in taste. Hence, less is needed in sweetening foods.

Another double sugar is *maltose*. It is an intermediate product of the digestion of starch in the body. It is also found in grains that have germinated and in products made from partly digested starch such as malted breakfast foods, malted milk and corn syrup. The sugar derived from corn starch is the simple sugar glucose.

Lactose is also a double sugar and is the only carbohydrate from an animal source that is used as a food. It is commonly called milk sugar. Although milk is the universal food of newborns, some infants cannot digest it because they lack sufficient amounts of lactase, the enzyme in the digestive tract that breaks down the lactose to glucose and galactose. The lack of this particular enzyme results in many adults not being able to tolerate milk. In those populations that habitually drink milk, the adults have more lactase. However, many individuals who are intolerant to lactose are able to drink limited amounts of milk or eat dairy products.

Starch is formed by combining many molecules of glucose. The starch molecule may contain as many as 300 to 400 groups of this simple sugar. Strangely, these large molecules, although composed of many sugar groups, do not have a sweet taste and are not soluble in water. Starch is the carbohydrate stored in roots, seeds, and tubers. In the plant, starch is stored in containers called granules that are covered with a cellulose-like substance. The starch granules of various plants differ in size and shape. When examined under the microscope these granules of starch identify the plants from which they were derived. When starch granules are treated by moist heat as in cooking, they absorb water, become swollen and rupture. The starch then forms a jelly-like or gluelike substance in the water. In this state it is more easily digested. Before starch can be used as a source of energy in the plant or in the human body, it must first be broken down into the simple sugar groups of which it is composed. Each starch molecule upon digestion yields many molecules of glucose. Dextrins, however, are more soluble than starch.

The chief food sources of starch are grains and, of course, products made from them such as breads, breakfast cereals, cakes and other baked goods and pastas. Other good sources of starch are legumes (beans and peas), certain tubers such as taro and cassava and root vegetables such as potatoes, yams and sweet potatoes.

Cellulose is also a polysaccharide. But it is less affected by digestion than starch. Cooking only softens cellulose. It is not digested by man. Therefore, it is not a source of available energy for humans. However, it is an energy source for ruminants (animals that chew the cud) because bacteria act on the cellulose prior to absorption in the animal's gut. Cellulose and *hemicellulose* (a closely-related complex carbohydrate) compose the structural part of plants such as the leaves, stems, roots, seed and peelings. Most of this fibrous material is not digested. Therefore, it acts as a source of bulk to the food residue in the intestine. The importance of fiber is receiving much study by the medical profession because of its possible preventive aspect in certain colon disorders.

Glycogen is another polysaccharide. It is sometimes called animal starch because it is the only polysaccharide stored in animal tissues. When the body needs sugar as glucose it breaks down glycogen. Then the glucose is burned to yield energy. This carbohydrate is an immediate source of fuel for all animals. Glucose is the only sugar stored in substantial amounts in the blood and tissue fluids. Only limited amounts of glycogen can be stored in the liver and muscles because it is rapidly used up during fasting and muscular activity. Therefore, only a very limited amount of carbohydrate is obtained from eating animal tissues.

Refined sugar and cornstarch are nearly pure carbohydrates. Refined sugar is about 99 percent carbohydrate and cornstarch about 90 percent. The rest of the weight is water. White rice and white flour are about 80 percent starch. They also contain small amounts of protein. However, whole-grain cereals have more protein and less starch. Dried peas and beans are about 20 percent protein and about 60 percent starch. Soybeans are an exception. They contain less starch and more protein. Legumes and whole grains contain certain minerals and vitamins also and are considered good sources of fiber. Starchy roots such as taro and cassava (manioc) serve as chief sources of carbohydrates in the South Pacific and certain parts of Africa. However, these have little protein, minerals or vitamins.

Table sugar, honey, candies, cakes, jams, jellies, syrups and dried fruits such as dates, figs, prunes, raisins, etc., are foods with a high sugar content—as high as 60 to 99 percent sugar. Fresh fruits contain from 9 to 23 percent sugar; soft drinks about 8 percent sugar. Fruits and soft drinks may contribute appreciable amounts of energy or calories if consumed in considerable quantities.

Grains such as wheat, corn, rice, rye and barley are rich in starch (about 50 to 85 percent). Cooked cereals, potatoes and legumes may contain about 10 to 20 percent carbohydrate. Cooked rice, pastas and sweet potatoes contain about 20 to 32 percent carbohydrate.

Carbohydrate-rich foods provide an economical source of energy for the body. At the same time, many of them furnish some protein, minerals and vitamins. Carbohydrates as sugars add flavor to foods and are important in food preservation but should be used in limited amounts as they provide little or no other nutrients.

CARBOHYDRATES QUIZ

Carbohydrates—a word we hear constantly in connection with dieting. How much do you know about this basic nutrient? Try the quiz below.

1. Carbohydrates are:
   A. The major source of energy in the diet
   B. A sure way to put on weight
   C. Only simple starch and sugar
   D. To be avoided at all costs

2. Carbohydrates are found in:
   A. Oats, corn and rice
   B. Potatoes, peanuts, and soybeans
   C. Bread
   D. Candies, jams, and molasses

3. Carbohydrates contain:
   A. Lots of oxygen and very little carbon
   B. Carbon, hydrogen, and oxygen
   C. A lot of hydrogen and little carbon
   D. Hydrogen and oxygen always in the same proportion as in water

4. Carbohydrates provide:
   A. About 30% of the world's energy needs
   B. About 70% of the world's energy needs
   C. About 90% of the world's energy needs
   D. Very little of the world's energy needs

5. Carbohydrates help our bodies in certain specific ways:
   A. Assist in the digestion and assimilation of other foods
   B. Provide immediately available calories for energy
   C. Help regulate protein and fat metabolism
   D. Allow the body to manufacture some of the B-complex vitamins

ANSWERS:

1. A—Carbohydrates are the chief source of energy for all body functions and muscular exertion.
2. A, B, C, and D. Wheat, oats, corn, rice, potatoes, noodles, and soybeans provide starch in our diet along with other important nutrients. In fruits, candies, jams and syrups carbohydrates are found in the form of sugar.
3. B and D. All carbohydrates are made of the chemical elements carbon, hydrogen and oxygen. The hydrogen and oxygen are always in the same proportion as in water.
4. B. 70% of the world's energy needs comes from carbohydrates. Grains, potatoes, vegetables such as taro, beans, and peas, and sugar cane and sugar beets are major world carbohydrate sources.
5. A, B, C, and D. Carbohydrates are important to our bodies in many different ways. They are a super quick energy source, but care must be taken not to overindulge in refined carbohydrates such as white flour and white sugar and products made from them. Diets high in refined carbohydrates are usually low in vitamins, minerals, and cellulose, and may perpetuate any vitamin B deficiency an individual may have.

14

MINERALS

by Dr. Eppie Hartsuiker

"The Lord God formed man of dust from the ground, and breathed into his nostrils the breath of life; and man became a living being" (Gen. 2:7). Therefore, it is not surprising to note that some of the elements found in the soil are also found in the human body. These elements are called minerals and are essential nutrients in that they are needed to regulate important functions in the body. For instance, many vitamins cannot carry on their functions in the body without certain minerals.

While plants synthesize some of their own nutrients patterned after their genetic or hereditary make-up, they also obtain nutrients from the soil such as inorganic minerals. Man must replenish his minerals by eating these plants or the flesh of animals and/or their products which also obtained their mineral supply from plants or other animals.

Minerals differ from carbohydrates, proteins and fats in that they are inorganic elements, which means they contain no carbon and are not energy-producing nutrients. Therefore, like water and vitamins, they contain no calories. When any food is burned, all that is left is the ash—the total mineral content of the food.

For discussion, minerals may be grouped according to the amounts found in the body. The most abundant minerals are called *macrominerals*. These include *calcium, phosphorus, magnesium* and the three electrolytes—*sodium, potassium* and *chlorine*. *Sulfur* is a mineral found also in large quantities in the body but it is utilized in an organic form, unlike the other minerals. The rest of the 20 to 30 remaining minerals are found in very small amounts in the body and are called *microminerals* or *trace elements*. Some of these trace elements known to be essential for body functions are *cobalt, copper, fluorine, iodine, iron, manganese, molybdenum, selenium* and *zinc*. One that appears to be essential is *chromium*. The functions of some are not known such as *aluminum, arsenic, boron, bromine, cadmium, lead, nickel, silicon, strontium* and *vanadium*.

The Recommended Dietary Allowances for minerals by the Food and Nutrition Board are given in milligrams and micrograms. (A milligram is 1/1,000 of a gram and a microgram is 1/1,000,000 of a gram. To give an idea of these measurements, one-fifth of a teaspoon of sugar weighs one gram.) The board has also given a range of recommended intake for several of the trace elements because there is less information on which to base allowances. It cautions that since the toxic levels for many trace elements may be only several times the usual intakes, the upper levels for these minerals should not be exceeded on a regular basis.

Most minerals are found in commonly eaten foods such as meat, fish, seafood, poultry, eggs, milk and dairy products, fruits, vegetables (especially the dark green, leafy ones), legumes (beans and peas), whole grain cereals, wheat germ, brewer's yeast, nuts and nut butters, iodized salt and fluoridated water. Since only very small amounts of minerals are needed for health, it is not necessary to eat huge quantities of any one food for its mineral content. In fact, eating an excess of any trace element can be harmful. However, it is not likely that one would obtain a toxic level from food sources alone.

Today man has decreased his mineral intake by certain culinary and dietary practices: discarding the peelings and hulls of mineral-rich foods; throwing away the cooking water which contains the dissolved minerals; increasing the use of refined foods; not selecting mineral-rich foods.

The total amount of minerals found in the average adult weighs about six-and-a-half pounds. About one-half of this is calcium, the most abundant mineral in the body. Phosphorus weighs about one-fourth of the total weight of body minerals. The remaining macrominerals make up another one-and-a-half pounds and the 25-30 trace elements, mostly iron, weigh about one ounce.

We will discuss three macrominerals only—calcium, phosphorus and magnesium.

Calcium and Phosphorus

The skeleton and the teeth are made up mainly of three minerals—calcium, phosphorus and magnesium. But the minerals fluorine and manganese and vitamins A, C, and D are also involved in the formation of bones and teeth. Even protein is not excluded. The teeth and bones contain 99 percent of the calcium and 70 percent of the phosphorus in the body. Therefore, these two minerals are usually classed together. The calcium to phosphorus ratio is 2:1 which is usually constant. Any marked change in one will cause a change in the other.

Bone is the supporting or structural part of the body. It is a good source of calcium which the body may call upon to keep the level of this mineral in the blood at a constant level. This is regulated by the two hormones (chemical messengers) parathyroid hormone and calcitonin, along with vitamin D. Throughout life bone is always being formed and dissolved. This action slows down with aging. In later years of life the dissolving process takes on a more prominent role so that more bone is lost than is being made. This accounts for the more frequent bone fractures in the elderly than among the young. This is thought to be a so-called normal process which usually begins in the fifties in both men and women. However, it appears to progress twice as fast in women as in men. Therefore, *calcium is an important nutrient* for the elderly, along with vitamin D.

Calcium is needed to clot blood, for the contraction of muscles, normal heart function, the normal transmission of the nerve impulse to perform work and the cementing function of various membranes.

Calcium is absorbed from the intestine by a method called *active transport*. This means it moves into the body by a process requiring energy. Vitamin D is needed also to ensure good absorption and utilization of both calcium and phosphorus in the diet. However, not all of the calcium obtained from food is absorbed. The normal amount is about 20-30 percent. This depends upon the dietary intake and the amount needed by the body. But a continuous intake of an excessive amount of calcium in the diet will cause most of it to be excreted in the feces. There are some dietary substances which influence the absorption of calcium from the intestine. Phytic acid and oxalic acid are such substances. They decrease the absorption of calcium by forming insoluble salts in the intestine. Swiss chard, beet greens, spinach and rhubarb contain oxalic acid. However, these foods are not believed to affect the calcium utilization of other foods eaten at the same time. Therefore, they are usually not considered to be foods to be avoided since they contain other important nutrients. However, the leaves of the rhubarb plant contain a high concentration of oxalic acid along with some other harmful substances. Therefore, the leaves should not be eaten at any time. Whole wheat and other whole grain cereals contain phytic acid which binds the calcium so that it is not absorbed. But some groups of people have been known to ingest high intakes of phytic acid as whole wheat, causing a loss of more calcium than is ingested, and yet appear to be in good health. It may be that the body makes some type of adjustments under certain circumstances. This brings into mind what the psalmist said about God taking into consideration where a man is born in making judgment upon that man (see Ps. 87:6).

For those who are unable to tolerate regular milk because of a lactase deficiency which produces gas, cramps and diarrhea, the substitution of buttermilk and yogurt will provide excellent sources of available calcium. Also, a fairly new product called acidophilus milk provides adequate amounts of calcium without the intolerance symptoms.

Phosphorus combines readily with carbohydrates, proteins and fats. Besides its functions in bones and teeth, it is a mineral needed for reproduction, for the transmission of the traits of heredity, for cell division and the synthesis of protein in the cells as well as others.

The diet will probably provide enough phosphorus if the calcium requirement of 800 milligrams per day for adults is met. However, additional amounts are needed during pregnancy and lactation. There are varying allowances for children, depending on age.

An excellent food source of calcium is milk. One cup of milk furnishes about 280 milligrams of calcium. Therefore three cups of milk daily will provide the day's requirement of calcium for an adult. Other good to fair sources of calcium are milk products, greens (collard, dandelion, kale, mustard and turnip), other vegetables, some fruits and nuts and most of the legumes (beans and peas).

Good food sources of phosphorus are milk and milk

products, legumes, nuts (especially peanuts and brazil nuts), oatmeal and other whole grain cereals, eggs, meats, fish and fowl. If a diet contains adequate amounts of protein, it will provide enough phosphorus.

The level of protein in the diet has a marked influence on the excretion of calcium in the urine. The higher the level of protein intake the higher the excretion of calcium in the urine. However, not all the data is in concerning the effect of high protein and low calcium intakes as far as calcium retention is concerned.

The transport of calcium takes place whenever the body needs it. Therefore, it is most active when the needs of the body are greatest, such as during pregnancy and lactation or when the amount of calcium supplied by the diet is limited, hence the importance of vitamins for mothers and growing children.

Magnesium

The normal body contains about an ounce of magnesium. It functions along with calcium and phosphorus to form bone and teeth. It is also important for the heart, nerves and muscles. It is necessary for the normal regulation of body temperature and the synthesis of protein.

Alcoholics may have low levels of magnesium, but average people seldom suffer from a deficiency because it is widely available in foods. The National Research Council recommends a magnesium allowance of 300-400 milligrams daily for adults, increasing to 450 milligrams during pregnancy and lactation. Amounts vary with age in infancy and childhood.

It is found in largest quantity in nuts, whole grains, legumes, and in green leafy vegetables because it is part of the structure of chlorophyll (the green pigment of leaves).

It acts as a catalyst for a number of functions in the body. (By definition a catalyst is a substance that initiates or accelerates a chemical reaction but is not consumed or changed permanently by it.) Magnesium is best known for its role in the transmission of the nerve impulse which leads to a contraction of a muscle.

About 40 percent of dietary magnesium is absorbed. A diet high in calcium increases the need for dietary magnesium because both of these minerals compete for the same places in the intestinal cells which transport these minerals. The absorption of magnesium is better in an acid medium and is inhibited by the presence of oxalic and phytic acids. Most of the magnesium in the body is distributed in bone and muscle. But it is found in blood, spinal fluid, heart and liver. It is involved in the utilization of carbohydrates as energy, protein synthesis and other functions requiring enzymic action.

A deficiency of magnesium has not been clearly defined in humans. This is because it is difficult to produce a deficiency state in man experimentally. A deficiency of magnesium is sometimes seen in alcoholism, in diseases of the liver such as liver cirrhosis, in conditions where there is an absorption problem in the intestine such as in sprue, in diabetic acidosis, in severe vomiting, in the long use of fluids given by other means than by mouth which do not contain magnesium and in the use of agents to increase the output of urine. Symptoms seen in a deficiency state include a change in the personality of the individual, spasms of the muscles without apparent cause, trembling, twitching of the muscles and delirium. For an individual who may have low levels of magnesium, it may be dangerous to give large amounts of calcium other than by mouth or to administer parathyroid hormone or vitamin D because there will be a tendency toward hardening of the soft tissues by deposits of calcium.

High levels of magnesium in the blood may be due to taking laxatives too frequently which contain magnesium or ingesting magnesium-containing drugs such as antacids.

The condition produces extreme thirst, excessive warmth, drowsiness, nerve irritability and exceedingly rapid contractions or twitching of the muscle fibers of the wall of the upper chamber of the heart called fibrillation. This causes the beat of the lower chamber of the heart to become disrupted. Death can occur if the normal rhythm of the heart is not reestablished. In the early states it can be corrected with the use of a substance called calcium gluconate.

The best and safest way to ensure an adequate intake of all the minerals is to eat a variety of foods from meal to meal and from day to day. This is God's way.

15

YOU CAN HAVE MORE ENERGY

by Willa Vae Bowles

Would you like for planet Earth to stop and let you off until you get rested and ready to *go* again? Do you often wonder why you are so tired when the day is yet so young? Or do you only wish you had energy like some of your friends?

When your energy level is low, you can't accomplish much so you easily become discouraged and depressed. Read on—there is hope!

There are several causes of depletion of energy. You cannot separate the functions of the spirit, mind and body. Each affects the others. I will give you some *nutritional* helps to give quick energy for times of need. But truthfully, the problem should be analyzed for the cause. Energy is an effect. Where is the energy leak?

It could be spiritual: Breaking God's laws and avoiding repentance to receive forgiveness brings a sense of condemnation that will affect every area of one's life. Forgiving yourself and all others and accepting God's love, mercy and forgiveness is the first step to a happy life enjoying perfect health.

Emotional: Repressed hatred, bitterness, unforgiveness, grudges and other negative emotions cause improper food digestion which leads to various organ or gland malfunctions that will soon sap a person's strength.

Lack of sleep: You can exist for a time without food, but water and sleep are a daily necessity for existence. Restful sleep is needed to maintain body metabolism. God created us to require sleep just as we do food, and the demand for sleep is as regular as that for food. During sleep the body, particularly the brain, has an opportunity to repair itself and build reserves of energy.

Stuffed colon: Your colon is a great sewage system, but by neglect or abuse it can become a cesspool. When it is clean and normal, you are well and energetic. When it stagnates, it will distill the poisons of decay, fermentation and putrefaction into the blood, which affects the brain and nervous system, organs and glands so that you are robbed of energy and become depressed. Noticeable symptoms of this problem could be a foul breath or a blemished facial skin. Controlled fasting, colonics or proper enemas are the quickest remedy. Dr. Christopher's lower-bowel herb combination or his red clover combination or just plain Aloe Vera Leaf capsules are a big help. The colon can be maintained by eating a raw apple before bedtime and eating papayas anytime. The enzymes in these fruits help digest and neutralize the toxic protein in the intestines.

Insufficient oxygen going through the lungs, bloodstream and to the brain brings on frequent times of sleepiness, inability to concentrate, dizziness and tiredness. Good breathing exercises and walking in fresh air will help. For a quick lift, while sitting or standing very straight inhale through your nose while slowly, silently counting to five. Hold your breath as you count to five or longer. Exhale slowly through your mouth. Continue for three minutes if possible. You can even do this while listening during a telephone conversation.

Inadequate liquids: Water is God's creation of moisture that nurtures all of life. Water makes up from 50 percent to 70 percent of your body and two-thirds of this amount is contained within the cells. It acts as a solvent to carry nutrients to the cells, transports waste products to be excreted by the kidneys and lungs, and is critical in the digestive process. Water also helps in regulating body temperature. There is no substitute for good drinking water!

Malabsorption of minerals, especially calcium, can cause a real imbalance that is a big energy leak to your system. Without minerals, vitamins cannot be adequately utilized by your body. One simple way of knowing if you have this problem is by checking your pH. If your pH is far off, you probably would benefit from taking Cal-Mag that you can purchase at health food stores. The heavier minerals such as iron, zinc, manganese and iodine are difficult to be absorbed by the body when deficient in calcium.

Extremely low or high blood sugar brings on severe exhaustion or fatigue. This is, in my opinion, the most common cause.

It has been proven that diabetics were once hypoglycemics (low blood sugar). All diabetics should be under the supervision of a competent physician. And all low blood sugar victims need help too! Many studies show how many prisoners, mental patients, hyper children and behavior-problem people can be changed into well-adjusted, productive, happy people by proper diet and food supplements. Many of these people are merely suffering from low blood sugar. It is an abnormally low level of glucose (sugar) in the blood caused by too much sugar in the diet or tumors in the pancreas or some disorder in the liver that interferes with storage and release of sugar. A quick rise and fall of blood sugar can cause headache or mental confusion, temper outburst, or loss of will to live because of lack of energy to cope with responsibilities.

Correct the Area That Is the Cause

You cannot simply think or confess your way out of physical tiredness with no attention to your diet. But by feeding yourself full-of-faith thoughts and proper foods you will become energetic. Your whole life will improve dramatically when your body is surging with energy to cope with every situation. It takes energy to mentally see life in proper focus.

The best approach to the energy-leak dilemma is to correct the cause. You may need the help of a dear friend or minister. For your physical need, I suggest you seek the services of a doctor who practices holistic ideas, and a good nutritionist. A test evaluation could be made from your blood, urine and hair to see just what minerals and vitamins you lack. You may need a diet prepared especially for you to help your body get into perfect chemical balance.

Unless you have an allergy to certain foods, the following nutritional suggestions will give you a temporary boost in energy.

Eat three balanced meals and three or four snacks. Mid-morning and mid-afternoon snacks can be prepared and taken to work. The following should not add weight if you do not overeat at mealtime.

1. One-fourth fresh fruit or four ounces fruit juice with a few sesame, pumpkin or sunflower seeds.

2. One-half cup cottage cheese with some warm or cool lemonade.

3. Ten soy protein tablets that contain B complex and lecithin (Superpro is the brand I use) and some diluted fruit juice.

4. Salt-free V-8 juice and RyKrisp.

5. One-half large avocado seasoned with Vegit or Spike and eight almonds.

6. One tablespoon sesame seeds soaked in kefir milk. Chew well.

7. One-half papaya or one sour apple.

8. One piece melon in season.

9. Four ounces pineapple juice, one tablespoon Brewer's yeast, one tablespoon calcium gluconate, one tablespoon lecithin. Mix in blender or shake in jar. Will keep at room temperature for several hours.

10. Slice of natural cheese with cup of hot lemonade or herb tea.

11. Stone-ground wheat crackers and ricotta cheese.

12. One cold boiled egg seasoned with cayenne pepper and lemonade.

13. One-third cup sunflower seeds and tomato juice.

14. Dried apricots soaked in distilled water and rolled in unsweetened coconut or chopped nuts.

15. One cup plain yogurt sprinkled with two teaspoons Brewer's yeast and one teaspoon raw honey.

16. Piece of homemade candy using honey, molasses, pure maple syrup or carob as sweeteners.

17. Three Chlorella Pura tablets (a new product that is a whole food rich in protein, minerals, chlorophyll but has less than one calorie per tablet).

Keep your snacks interesting with variety. The energy-producing foods such as brewer's yeast, lecithin, wheat germ, protein powder or tablets, and vegetable or nut oils can be added to many snack creations.

All sugars, including honey, molasses, fructose and pure maple syrup, give quick energy, but in the majority of people they can cause the blood sugar to rise—just to fall—and leave you weaker than before.

Give Yourself a Mini-Tune-Up
Begin by being good to yourself in arranging a day or two for complete rest. During this time fast on fruit and/or vegetable juices. Take no vitamins, minerals or herbs. Do some good reading.

Too Busy to Cook?

Many "meals in a glass" can be prepared in your blender that will give quick energy. These may be used with a slice of whole-grain toast with butter or natural cheese for breakfast or with a mixed-vegetable salad for lunch. Remember variety is the key to getting many minerals and vitamins. Try for breakfast:

> 4 oz. skim milk or 1/2 cup yogurt
> 1/2 cup almonds
> 6 pitted dates (previously soaked in water)
> 1/4 cup unsweetened coconut
> 1 T. raw honey
> 1 tsp. blackstrap molasses
> 1 T. liquid corn oil
> 1 small banana
> 1/2 tsp. vanilla
> Ice as desired

Put all items in blender and blend until smooth. It's very filling and provides energy-producing nutrients.

Or try this one
6 oz. apricot nectar (or any other unsweetened fruit juice)

> 1 T. safflower oil
> 1 T. (heaping) Brewer's yeast
> 1 T. lecithin granules
> 1 T. calcium gluconate
> 1 tsp. raw honey

Blend in blender or shake in jar until smooth. Watch your energy soar. If you are extra weary, take a multi-vitamin/mineral plus a high-potency B complex and C.

Most Simple, Effective Energy Booster

Dr. G. K. Knowlton of Tulsa told me a very quick way to get immediate energy: Take 100 milligrams pantothenic acid with four ounces of fruit juice when you first begin to feel tired. The pantothenic acid will stimulate the adrenal glands while the fruit juice is bringing the blood sugar up. I have also found this to be successful in alleviating allergy symptoms.

Drinking coffee or soda pop made with sugar and eating pies, candy, cake and cookies give you a short perk-up in energy but suddenly let you down. You crave more sweets; it's a vicious circle. Why? Because you are stuffing yourself with empty calories with no nutrients to feed and maintain your body. And sugary foods burn up the B vitamins so that eventually you are very nervous, depressed, tense and irritable. Therefore, avoid all foods made with sugar. Otherwise you are sowing wind to reap a whirlwind.

Let the real you, your spirit, take control of your conscious mind to think only full-of-faith thoughts and dictate your food intake.

You have only one body, and it's got to last your lifetime.

16

BEAUTIFUL SKIN NATURALLY

by Dr. Susan Smith Jones

Your skin will be the first to give away your deep, dark secrets. If you've been neglecting your health and are under extra tension and pressure, if you haven't been able to sleep well because of worries, your skin will let the world know.

The skin is the largest single organ of the body and comes in many colors, textures and patterns. "Imagine a material that is water-proof, like tarpaulin, yet can let out water and oil, that can protect like a suit of armor, and yet is infinitely sensitive to touch, that remains firm yet is more flexible than rubber. It is also a beautiful material—whether pink and white, brown, black or yellow," according to consultant Elliott M. Goldwag, Ph.D.

Weighing in at approximately six pounds, the skin is about one-eighth of an inch thick, varying at different areas of the body. Beauty is in the eye of the beholder, but all we ever see of one another is skin surfaces and hair. The skin is continually growing from within, creating new cells that push their way outward. The skin on the palm of your hand renews every 24 hours. Yet the skin, perhaps more than any other part of the body, tells the world how we feel mentally and physically as well as how we care for and respect our bodies. American Indians used to diagnose body ailments by the lines in the face. The face is certainly the one area on the body which is unrestrained at keeping secrets.

The skin of an adult covers a surface area of about 18 to 20 square feet. It is well supplied with a variety of glands, blood vessels and nerves, and consists of three distinct layers: the epidermis (which is composed of four sublayers), the dermis, and the subcutaneous fat. The dermis layer relies on the protein *collagen* to keep it in mint condition by acting as a supporter and major building block of the skin. *Elastin*, also a protein, along with collagen gives the skin its supple, elastic quality.

Functions of the Skin

Two million pores cover our body's surface and function as an efficient cooling system. Any exercise can raise internal temperature to seven degrees above normal. The body dissipates that excess heat through perspiration, which evaporates on the skin.

Besides cooling and protecting the body, the skin also serves as a sense organ. The fetus probably receives most sensations through the skin. From the moment of birth, humans require touching and physical affection as much as food.

Yet what is so amazing is that no two people on earth have identical skin formation—not even twins—as demonstrated in the science of fingerprinting. What's more, the fingerprints of the right hand even differ from those of the left hand. A woman's fingerprints, in fact, tend to have more arches and fewer swirls than a man's.

Sun and the Skin

Without the sun, there would be no life. Too much sun and there's lifeless skin, which calls to mind the venerable adage, "everything in moderation." "Let your moderation be known unto all men" (Phil. 4:5, *KJV*). Let this be your guide in regard to sun exposure.

The sun brings more people outdoors, which means more exposure of the skin's surface to the sun. What a paradoxical situation this can be. On one side of the coin, the sun is the body's most effective/efficient and least expensive source of vitamin D, appropriately termed the "sunshine" vitamin because the action of the sun's ultraviolet rays activates a form of cholesterol, which is present in the skin, converting it to vitamin D. Most of the body's needs for vitamin D can be met by sufficient exposure to sunlight, according to John Kircshmann in *Nutrition Almanac*, and from the eating of small amounts of food—fish liver oils, egg yolks, milk, butter, salmon, sprouted seeds, mushrooms, and sunflower seeds.

On the other side of the coin, many feel that a deep golden tan is the mark of the leisure class, portraying health and beauty. The sun does have some beneficial effects such as clearing up acne, relaxing tired muscles, and creating a positive psychological effect on people. Too much of this good thing, however, can be the skin's worst enemy.

Earlier generations knew the wisdom of protecting the skin against the strong light. They would have agreed with Virginia Castleton's remarks in *The Handbook of Natural Beauty,* to the effect that sunlight, rather than the aging process, is largely responsible for senile skin. This is obvious in many young people—especially those who are addicted to sun baking.

In a recent interview with Barbara Elleck, of the New Beginning Salon in Pasadena, California, many interesting facts about the sun and the skin were discussed.

She pointed out that heavy doses of sunlight can dry and age the skin of both men and women and it's difficult to say what is too much sun. "Overexposure to the sun can break down the collagen and elastin components of the skin, causing loss of moisture, flexibility and tautness. The best proof of this is to observe the skin after a few years of constantly maintaining a suntan."

Similarly, I chatted with beauty specialist and author Trenna Sutphen from Scottsdale, Arizona, who concurs, "Too much sun will cause the skin to line before its time, followed by premature sagging. The sun damage is rapid and accumulative. Those rays can be damaging even on gray winter days."

Aside from the leathery, sagging, weathered look, the sun can also cause dark patches and scaly gray growths, called *keratoses*, that are sometimes precancerous. The most dangerous effect of too much sun is the potential for skin cancer. In 1977 350,000 people in the United States contracted skin cancer. That's about half of all cases of cancer reported.

According to the American Cancer Society, almost all skin cancer is considered sun-related. Fortunately, it is 95 percent curable. Watch for such signs as an eruption or sore that doesn't heal but continues to bleed and then scab and bleed again. A dark spot or freckle that grows larger should be checked by a physician, as should any change in a wart, sore, or a scaly, reddened patch on the skin.

Here are some pointers I have gleaned for sun protection:

• Bald men should cover their heads with sunscreen if they go hatless.

• Skiers need sunscreen more than swimmers. Snow and ice reflect about 90 percent of the sun's ultraviolet radiation while dry sand reflects only about 40 percent.

• Sunscreens work better when applied 30 minutes to one hour before exposure to the sun.

• Clouds consist of water vapor easily penetrated by sunlight. Hazy days are equally deceptive. A protective lotion should be worn despite the overcast sky.

● Time in the water is considered time in the sun.

My advice is that whatever your relationship with the sun: an occasional acquaintance, intimate friend, or easy prey, enjoy its warmth and life-giving properties, but don't lose your skin.

Nutritional Life-Giving Properties

The wholesomeness of our skin will be affected by our diet. Ask yourself if your nutritional pattern measures up. Reduce or eliminate most animal fats and hard oils from the diet, but maintain a normal intake of liquid vegetable oils. Chocolate in any form should be avoided, and sweets reduced or eliminated. Eat as many things raw as possible and steam vegetables until barely done. This retains flavor and the vitamins. Use herbs and seasonings lavishly; they add flavor and eye appeal. Use yogurt and buttermilk as a base for salad dressings instead of sour cream and mayonnaise. Use tomato juice instead of catsup, carob powder instead of cocoa, and broth instead of oil to sauté foods in a teflon skillet.

Some other important points for more beautiful skin are to eat moderately, carefully, watching not to stuff yourself. Cleanse your system by "fasting" periodically on fresh fruit and vegetable juices. As nutritional insurance, I recommend taking vitamin and mineral supplements which will have a positive effect on your skin as well as your general well-being.

Exercise and the Skin

Exercise is a terrific way to cleanse the body and clean out the pores. The exercise must be endurance-type activity which increases the heart rate and causes perspiration. After this type of exercise, walking, running, cycling and jumping rope, the skin takes on a beautiful, natural glow that no make-up artist could duplicate.

For Beautiful Looking Skin
Vitamin C is essential to include daily in the diet as it's one of the building blocks of collagen which holds our cells and the tissue together.

Positive Thoughts
Nutrition of the mind and spirit is also extremely important. Harboring feelings of fear, doubt, worry, guilt and criticism will result in negative-looking skin. Beautiful skin is a product of body, mind and spirit—total health.

17

HOW TO TREAT ALLERGIES

by Willa Vae Bowles

As a child *allergies* was an uncommon word to me. No one in my family or close circle of friends suffered the malady. During my college years a few classmates sneezed and blew their noses often, saying they hated the "hay fever" season. I thought they merely had a cold.

Then at the age of 28, I suddenly itched deep down between the eyes where I could not scratch! Soon came the sneezing, watery eyes, excess mucus and all the misery. Finally one night I could not breathe unless in a sitting position; this was the deciding factor for me to consult medical help.

I sought the services of a highly-recommended allergy specialist in the area who gave me the skin test for many pollens, food, animals, etc. My only enemies were three types of grass for which he prescribed injections twice weekly for one year. My symptoms promptly diminished and I faithfully took the injections, anticipating no allergies the next season. However, the next spring I suffered much worse than before.

Another series of tests was administered to discover that

I no longer was allergic to those three grasses but now had allergic reactions to redwood trees, several flowers and foods. Another series of injections and pills began!

Enough of this nonsense. I prayed for guidance and help! Then I was led to an osteopath named Dr. Marion van Ronk who tried to correct my diet and gave me food supplements. After questioning me about my eating habits and past life, she explained that the loss of my baby and husband, a miscarriage and a few other traumatic experiences all within one year had brought about my first allergy symptoms the following year. Evidently my adrenal glands were totally exhausted. I began an education in foods and supplements and helped myself build a strong resistance so that I gradually overcame all allergies except to a few foods and house-cleaning agents.

Allergy Symptoms

It is generally agreed that stress, tension, shocks, fright, severe fatigue, extreme anger or other emotional disturbances can cause or aggravate symptoms of allergies. This is because the adrenal glands become depleted when they excrete their vital hormone to aid the sympathetic nervous system to meet the demands of these emotions. The resulting underactivity of the adrenal glands means a deficiency of the hormones which serve the purpose of neutralizing wastes. This can cause a loss of protein, potassium, phosphorous, calcium and vitamin C. Also, when a person is under abnormal stress or displaying extreme emotions, he usually is not eating balanced meals. Without doubt what he does eat is not properly digested, which also causes adrenal exhaustion.

Allergy is among the most common of all human suffering. It is a reaction to a particular substance in a person sensitive to that substance. Innumerable substances can cause reactions, including pollens, foods, artificial coloring and flavorings, food preservatives, chlorine and fluorine in drinking water, dust, animal dander, drugs, cosmetics, toilet articles, dyes, chemicals, plants and fabrics.

A wide variety of symptoms is caused by allergies. Since many of these symptoms are also caused by other physical problems, the diagnosis is often difficult to establish. The most common allergies are hay fever, asthma, hives, skin rash, eczema, severe headaches, contact dermatitis such as poison ivy, dizziness, nausea, eye and eyelid conditions and digestive upsets.

My personal opinion is that the most prevalent allergy is to white sugar and bleached flour, and it is probably caused by the chemicals used in processing. However, it is very difficult to prove this or to convince people that this is their problem. A large percentage of our population is hypo- or hyperglycemic simply because white sugar and flour is poison to them. I feel that many unexplained physical ailments will someday be proven to be an allergy to man-processed foods and air pollution. The safest rule is to eat foods as near as possible to the way God created them!

Food Allergies

People may be sensitive to one or more foods. The most frequent allergy-producing are the common foods such as milk, eggs, wheat, fish, and nuts. This is unfortunate because these are also essential foods. The best immediate remedy for the annoying food allergy symptoms is to avoid that food and all dishes containing that food. I suppose that there is no food that does not produce allergies in someone. However, it is usually the protein in the food that causes the most serious problems; and often when the person takes a good digestant containing HCl and enzymes, he can tolerate the food. Eating more fruits and vegetables or drinking their juice will provide many enzymes.

If you do not know just which food is causing your

problem, you can try the mono diet. Eat only one food for your entire meal and see if you have a reaction. By the process of elimination you will discover your enemy.

Artificially colored, prepared and preserved foods should be considered "a little poison." The small amount of chemicals added cannot be proven to be harmful, but they all add up to health problems for those whose tolerance is low. Occasionally eating foods containing sodium nitrate, sodium nitrite, monosodium glutamate, benzoate of soda, BHA, BHT, sulphur dioxide and other chemicals will do no harm, but eating foods containing these every day often induces a physical system that has a low resistance to disease.

Avoid fruits that are seedless because they have been cross-bred to reproduce without any pits or seeds. These are also usually chemically fertilized and treated to grow and ripen rapidly. This is contrary to God's creative laws. These fruits are not as rich in minerals.

Avoiding white sugar and flour often eliminates the allergy symptoms to other foods. Excessive sugar, including honey, molasses, and alcohol, interferes with the absorption and metabolism of calcium as well as the important B vitamins. Experiments have proven that with babies many skin rashes, infections, eye conditions, excessive mucus, upset stomach and nervous problems improve just as soon as sugar or syrup is eliminated from their formulas. It is always best for mothers to breast-feed their babies the first year.

For perfect digestion of your food you need many enzymes, and each one is specific; that is, each acts on certain types of food substances and brings about a chemical reaction. There are certain enzymes in the mouth, others in the stomach and still more in the small intestine. The liver and pancreas have an important part in the production of enzymes. Your saliva contains an enzyme which acts on starch to convert it into sugar. Pepsin and hydrochloric acid (HCl) act to break down protein in the stomach. Milk is coagulated in the stomach by the action of HCl, pepsin and other substances such as rennin. And on and on. Pancreatic enzymes are concerned with the digestion of carbohydrates, fats and proteins as well as fat-soluble vitamins A, D, E, and K.

Because enzymes are living cells, they are sensitive to heat and cold. Consequently heating food too hot destroys them and cold temperatures will suspend their activity. Enzymes work best at body temperature. When enzymes ordinarily present in food are destroyed by cooking, the body is required to manufacture more. A large share of these enzymes have to be manufactured in the pancreas; if we eat too much overcooked or processed food, we over-work the pancreas to produce more enzymes and this can upset the digestion of proteins, fats and other nutrients. Thus, we do not have sufficient antibodies and often suffer allergy symptoms. This is why we need some fresh, raw food daily so that we will supply our body with natural enzymes and not overwork our pancreas.

Building Resistance to Allergies

Rid your body of toxins and you will ease allergic symptoms. After you detoxify, you can build up allergy fighters or antibodies in the bloodstream. How? Let us first consider the largest gland, the *liver*. Every vein from every part of the digestive tract empties into the liver through the portal vein. The proteins, sugars, and starches absorbed by the blood vessels of the stomach, by the small and large intestines and by the pancreas are brought to the liver in the blood. Bile is continually produced by your liver to assist in the breakdown and absorption of food fats. Your liver takes sugar from the blood and stores it as *glycogen* which is quickly converted back to sugar when needed by your body.

Your liver also produces *urea* which is taken by the blood to the kidneys for excretion. Your liver performs some 300 functions; one vital activity it does is the formation of many *antibodies* to counteract or fight infection or any kind of invaders or toxins in the body. Allergy victims usually catch cold or any other contagious disease easily because of a low antibody count.

To build antibodies you must absorb sufficient protein. Many people are not properly digesting and absorbing protein benefits due to a toxic liver. Wrong eating has made the body become a storehouse of accumulated, uneliminated poisons. The best way to detoxify and at the same time purify the bloodstream is to fast and rest for a few days. You must detoxify your liver before starting to rebuild your body. There are several beneficial cleansing fasts.

Dr. Beiler's Fast

If you do not have any symptoms of a serious disease, you might enjoy the late Dr. Beiler's fast which has helped many to transfer from a life of chronic fatigue to a life of much energy and strong resistance to disease. He suggests that you daily cook (but not overcook) in about two quarts of distilled water: zucchini, celery, string beans, an onion and a handful of parsley. Put these cooked vegetables, water and all, in a blender and make a vegetable broth. You drink 4 to 6 ounces of this broth every hour for two to four days. During this time you must stay in bed for a complete rest. Do not read anything exciting or watch TV. Listen to soft, relaxing music or listen to good teaching tapes that help you relax. It is important that you do not exert yourself. An enema should be taken each day to prevent toxins from reentering the bloodstream from the colon wall.

This fast will help to cleanse and rebuild the liver. If the liver is not working properly, all the minerals, vitamins and other nutrients you consume are not properly metabolized and instead of nutrients they become poisons in your body.

You may wish to cleanse your liver, kidneys and bowels following Dr. Donsbach's instructions. His booklets on many subjects (all contain the fast outline) are available at Health Food Stores.

Another quick liver cleanse: Make a punch using the juice of 6 lemons, 6 grapefruit and 12 oranges and 2 quarts of distilled water. Upon arising, take 1 tablespoon of epsom salts dissolved in 4 ounces of distilled water. Repeat in 30 minutes. Repeat again in 30 minutes (total 3 doses). Two hours later begin drinking a glass of the punch every 1/2 hour until all is consumed. If you feel hungry toward evening, you may have more grapefruit juice and some celery. Before going to bed, take an enema using two quarts of tepid water and the juice of one lemon. You may eliminate taking the epsom salts but continue taking the punch for two more days for a thorough cleansing. Even though the best results come when you are relaxed, you do not have to stay in bed the full time on this fast.

Poultry and Grape Juice Fast

If you simply cannot stay in bed and liquid fast, you may wish to do the Poultry and Grape Juice Fast. For one or two full days, your only intake will be skinned, baked white meat of chicken or turkey and concord grape juice diluted half with distilled water. (If you are diabetic, check with your doctor first.) God created grapes for man's beneficial use. Throughout the Bible grapes were eaten and one of the promises of blessing was that the vines would be fruitful. Grapes contain many minerals and vitamins with an easily digestible form of carbohydrate. The acid in the grape juice makes the meat easier to digest and not overwork the liver. Thus, you will be helping to revitalize your liver and build necessary antibodies to fight allergens or any other unwanted invaders.

After your liver is cleansed, the other glands and organs will respond more quickly to the nutrients in your foods and supplements for restoration. As a result of the cleanse, you may find the allergy symptoms have vanished. Great! But usually the *adrenal function* has been impaired. Foods rich in B-complex and additional pantothenic acid (B5), pyridoxine (B6) and vitamin C together with an adequate supply of all minerals will help rebuild the adrenals. Many nutritionists use a glandular formula containing dehydrated adrenal tissue, liver and spleen tissue, with vitamins A, C, B1, B2, B3, B5, B6 and zinc.

Pantothenic acid is absolutely essential to the production of antibodies. Royal jelly made by the honey bee is the richest source known. It is important to remember that anytime you are taking a large dose of any B vitamin such as pantothenic acid, you need the B-complex to help assimilation. Brewer's yeast and desiccated liver are rich sources which can be added to fruit or vegetable juice or meatloaf and casseroles. Soy flour, sunflower seeds and sesame seeds also contain appreciable amounts of pantothenic acid.

When the pituitary gland is not getting sufficient magnesium, it fails in its functional control over the adrenals, which allows the adrenals to overproduce adrenalin. The more protein you eat, the more your need for magnesium for the metabolization process. Fresh green vegetables, raw wheat germ and almonds are good sources. And, of course, it is available in supplement form should your test show a significant deficiency.

Ordinary salt is often used to stimulate the adrenal glands; however, you should not use excessive salt unless your tests show that you have a low salt level in your body.

If You Have an Allergy Attack
1. Avoid the cause.
2. Chew 200 mg. pantothenic acid with 4 ounces fruit

juice. If this does not give relief, try adding 1,000 mg. vitamin C. (For low-blood-sugar people, too much vitamin C can overstimulate the already overworking pancreas; therefore, it is suggested that you take high dosages only as needed.)

3. If pantothenic acid is not available, eat a small amount of dark raw honey and honeycomb.

4. Vitamin C has been used temporarily in dosages of 2,000 to 5,000 mg. daily to relieve symptoms of asthma, pollen-induced problems and a clogged nose.

Overcoming Allergy Problems

God never repairs a damaged cell. He allows the body to slough it out and replaces it with a live, vital cell. Our bodies are made up of countless cells. All tissue is made up of individual cells. Our goal is to constantly be creating new, live cells to replace those that are routinely being sloughed out. The cause of allergies and all other diseases is a mineral and vitamin deficiency. Actually it is a mineral deficiency because your body has a difficult time absorbing vitamins when the necessary minerals are inadequate. So the first thing I suggest is that you have a urine and/or blood test as well as send your hair sample to the lab for a mineral analysis. While waiting for the results of this analysis, go on the detoxification fast. Your lab tests will reveal the critical levels of vital minerals used by your body as well as show toxic elements being absorbed from environmental contact (such as too much lead in your body from car exhaust fumes).

Your body contains about seven times more calcium than any other mineral, and it is imperative it have some of the several kinds of calcium so the liver can manufacture its billions of enzymes to keep the food properly absorbing and building new cells. When you are calcium deficient, your body may start leeching it from your bones and teeth. People with allergy problems are calcium and trace mineral deficient. Maybe just a few minerals will put the body into balance. And, medically speaking, there are a few people who will always have to avoid some foods, cosmetics or household cleaning items because their bodies reject them.

18

KEEP HEALTHY WITH EXERCISE

by Dan Kubelka

How many of your friends have survived to retirement age? Wouldn't you like your retirement years to be a rewarding experience? No matter what your plans are for the years to come, they will depend on your good health.

Periodic medical checkups, proper diet and exercise are of paramount importance in maintaining good health. Before exercise is begun, however, a thorough physical examination including a stress test should be performed. This examination can help to determine levels of fitness, possible underlying diseases, contradictions to specific exercises, and the efficiency of the heart and vital organs.

After you have been given clearance by your doctor to begin an exercise program, you should remember the words *gradual* and *slow*. It took some time for you to get out of shape, so it will take some time to get back into shape. In order for you to understand what is happening to your body, let us analyze it.

The body is a machine that burns carbon and releases carbon dioxide, water, and energy. It operates some 639 muscles which move the body about. The efficiency of the body is determined by the ease with which fuel and oxygen are delivered to the cell. This delivery system incorporates the use of the blood vessels as pathways and the heart as pump.

The heart is actually two pumps. This double pump supplies blood to the lungs to replenish its oxygen supply, while at the same time it pumps oxygen and fuel to all parts of the body. It is by far the strongest muscle in the body, stopping only when you have a heart attack or die. It can pump from one-and-a-half to eight gallons of blood per minute while forcing it through some 60,000 miles of blood vessels. Many blood vessels are so small that 50 would be needed to equal the diameter of a hair.

It has been established that for every pound of fat, 4,000 capillaries are needed to nourish it. Imagine, if you are only 10 pounds overweight, the heart must pump blood through eight more miles of vessels. The saga doesn't end here. If the heart is out of shape and your arteries are hardening and accumulating plaque on the interior walls, the heart can have difficulty functioning.

In order for the heart to function, however, it must have oxygen. Oxygen is supplied through the blood by the lungs. The lungs can be affected by many afflictions, but one of the most common irritators is smoke. Carbon monoxide, which is a common ingredient in smoke, is readily absorbed by the red blood cells that carry oxygen. By smoking you are depriving your body of precious oxygen that is needed for all of your body functions.

By now you might be wondering if there is any hope for you and your time-ravaged body. You may think you are too old to change. You are never too old to begin to drop old habits.

Doctors and researchers have come to realize that many infirmities of old age are often due to inactivity. It is more important than ever as you grow older to maintain a degree of fitness through exercise.

Current research indicates that consistent exercise reduces the effects of the aging process. Some researchers postulate that regular exercise may retard the deposition of lipids in the arterial wall (a cause of many heart attacks). Exercise can also virtually eliminate many aches and pains that are due to poor circulation.

Exercise forces the blood to circulate. When flexing and extending muscles, many blood vessels are expanded and contracted, causing a pumping and flushing action of the blood. Waste products that may have pooled in a given area due to poor circulation are hence carried away in the bloodstream and nutrients replete with a fresh oxygen supply are pumped in.

Parts of the body that have been cold all the time can be warmed up as a result of consistent exercise.

Arm Rotations

A stimulating exercise that is good to do at the beginning, during, or at the end of an exercise workout is arm rotations. This exercise promotes circulation in the shoulders, where many people are often plagued with soreness.

Stand or sit erect. Raise straight arms to shoulder's height by your sides and rotate them clockwise for 10 seconds. Stop! Rotate counterclockwise for 10 seconds. You can vary the rotation of your arms by bendng your arms.

As your body and you become more accustomed to exercise, you may wish to join in other sporting activities. The parks and recreation department in your city probably has a myriad of physical activities. For the avid track enthusiast, there is the Senior Olympics held every year in different parts of the country. Some people in their eighties compete in these games. There are also senior masters' tournaments in golf and tennis as well as other sports that are held throughout the United States.

Push Aways

With advancing years and lack of exercise we may find the underside of our arms to be sagging and the muscles lacking in tone. A good exercise to alleviate this problem and add tone to the muscle is the push away.

Stand about two-and-a-half feet away from the wall. Place your palms shoulder's width apart about chest high on the wall. Gradually bend your arms, keeping your legs straight, until your chest is almost touching the wall, then extend your arms. Repeat this exercise 10 times. As you become stronger, work up to doing three sets of 10 repetitions.

Incline Push-Ups

If you feel the push away is too easy for you, the incline push-up is a little more advanced. It is also a good lead-up exercise to the most advanced form, the push-up.

Kneel down. Place palms on the floor shoulder's width apart, approximately three feet in front of the knees. Bend the arms and, keeping the back straight, lower the torso until your chest almost touches the floor. Extend your arms. Repeat the exercise keeping the back straight at all times. Do 10 repetitions and, as strength improves, increase the sets to three.

Knee-Ups

Sit on the floor with legs straight and hands on the floor slightly behind and away from your buttocks. Pull your knees toward your chest and try to hold them there for five seconds. Extend your legs and repeat the exercise 10 times or as often as you can. This exercise will work on your abdominal muscles as well as hip flexors. As your strength increases you may work up to two sets of 10 repetitions.

Squats

Although walking, jogging and running are great cardiovascular exercises that promote circulation, they don't develop the strength in the thighs that can be developed from the squat. This strength is vital in forestalling fatigue and enjoying the rigors of everyday life.

Stand with feet shoulder's width apart with heels resting on something one-and-a-half inches off the floor. With your arms by your side, gradually squat down until your thighs are almost parallel to the floor. Extend your legs and repeat the exercise 10 times. As your strength increases work up to three sets of 10 repetitions.

Book Curls

Your bicep muscles need exercise too. These muscles in your upper arm, when strengthened, allow you to perform your lifting chores with much greater ease and less fatigue. Weighted arm curls promote the strengthening of these muscles.

Pick up equal-weighted books in each hand. With your arms by your sides rotate your hands so that the books are facing the front, then keeping the elbows by your sides lift the books to your shoulders. Gradually lower the books to your sides again and repeat the exercise 10 times. As you increase in strength you can increase the repetitions to 15 and the sets to three. Do the curls slowly and concentrate on flexing the biceps.

Seated Towel Pulls

Strength in the shoulders and upper back tends to dissipate with age. To retard this loss of strength we need to exercise this portion of the body. The seated towel pull is an aid to developing strength in the shoulders and upper back.

Sit on the floor. Holding each end of a towel, bend your knees and place the towel over the bottoms of both feet.

While maintaining balance and still holding on to the towel, extend your legs. This is the starting position. While slowly bending the legs pull the two ends of the towel toward you, rolling your shoulders back as far as possible until you have pulled the towel in as far as you can. Repeat the exercise 10 times. As strength increases, do three sets of 10 repetitions. If balance is a problem, put a pillow slightly behind the buttocks.

There are many exercises that can be performed that will enhance your physique and retard the aging process that we have not mentioned. We hope that these will help get you started.

19

WALKING FOR HEALTH

by Dr. Charles Serritella

My enthusiasm for the art of walking began in New Jersey when I was a kid. In the thirties we formed hiking groups and on Sundays we would hike through the trails and forests of the northern part of the state. In 1935 Bernarr Macfadden, the physical culturist, began his annual two weeks Health Walks and I was able to take part in all but one of them. Beginning in 1937 I competed in walking races in the Northeast and in the Midwest, with the distances running from one mile to 31.1 miles (50,000 meters). Many of the races were National AAU championships. While a navy corpsman in World War II, attached to Sea Bees on shore duty in the British Isles, I was able to enjoy the beautiful scenery and excellent walking in England, Scotland and Wales. Here are some of my thoughts and experiences regarding the wonderful world of walking.

Health Benefits
A regular three-mile-daily walk enhances the efficiency of our cardiovascular and respiratory systems. Heart and

blood vessels are helped and blood pressure tends to become normalized. The lungs and entire respiratory tract are improved as well as organs, tissues and tissue cells. The brain can function better because of the accelerated removal of wastes from the blood and the influx of oxygen and other needed nutrients into the millions of individual brain tissue cells. This pattern follows with all of the trillion other tissue cells throughout the body, removing wastes and supplying oxygen. Digestion and elimination are also helped.

After a refreshing walk and a shower we are exhilarated for our daily tasks, and we're not nearly as pooped at the end of the day. Believe it or not, even our relations with others improve because we feel better. Here is a "high" without drugs or alcohol.

Foot Care

The importance of a good, comfortable pair of walking shoes cannot be overemphasized. The joggers' and runners' shoes on the market now are just fantastic. Find a pair that fits well and feels good to your feet. Most walkers wear a pair of sweat socks for comfort. With the right pair of shoes you will feel like you are almost floating along. Before and after walking be sure to do a few stretching exercises (described later).

If blisters develop, take good care of them. After bathing, cover them with Vaseline and a cushion of cotton covered with strips of adhesive tape and leave the bandage on a few days, even after bathing. Then open the edges of the blister with a sterilized needle, allowing as much of the fluid out as possible. Bandage again for a day or two with Vaseline, cotton and tape and allow the under skin to heal. Then trim away the outer skin, sterilize with Bactine or Merthiolate and bandage with a little Vaseline, cotton and tape until healed.

Exercises

Let's look at some exercises which will improve muscle strength, tone and flexibility to help your walking. My favorite one is to hold on to the back of a chair with your hands, standing back a few feet. Dip your pelvis forward toward the chair, to loosen the lower back. After several movements, stand erect with feet apart and do a pelvic twist slowly, first one way and then the other. Then raise up on your heels, lifting the toes as high as you can, and hold for a few seconds, stretching the back of the legs, the entire back, shoulders, arms and the neck. Place the toes down and rise on them, then repeat the procedure. Rising on the toes is a good exercise to give added bounce to your step. Repeat all procedures as many times during the day as you can manage. If you are a desk worker you will find these exercises refreshing. All the exercises should be performed slowly, without straining. My back patients like the movements and do them whenever they can find a few minutes to spare.

Before going to sleep, and in the morning prior to arising, pull the knees to the chest and slowly pump the lower legs up and down. This exercise will help to tighten the abdominal and lower back muscles and help keep the knees flexible. Slowly raise one leg upward as far as you can and then raise the other. Then raise both legs and lower. Another movement is to bend both legs toward the chest, straighten upward and then slowly lower. While on your back it is a good idea to do ankle exercises to achieve good flexibility to help avoid ankle sprains. Rotate ankles inwardly and then outwardly a few times, then bend downward and stretch upwards.

Stand with arms outstretched, rotate arms and shoulders one way and then the other. Put your head down and reach forward as high as you can, forward and backward. This helps to loosen the lower neck. A few push-ups or chin-ups will help strengthen the upper body.

Persons wishing to go on to a faster race walking stride of say 12-minute miles or better will need to learn to allow the pelvis to reach farther forward with each stride. This is "free distance." Race walkers use this hip-swinging style to cover more ground at a faster speed. It is noted that most women have easier swinging hips than most men. No doubt this is because they need extra flexibility of the pelvic musculature for childbirth. To achieve greater flexibility, slow and easy stretching exercises should be performed as often as possible. Stretch forward, sideward and backward as far as you can.

Trunk exercises are important for everyone as well as walkers to help avoid lower back strain. With feet apart and hands on hips bend forward, stretch backward, bend sideward left and right and then rotate slowly to the left and right. Don't underestimate the value of this simple but important exercise. Keeping the trunk flexible helps walking.

Walking Style

It is my belief that a modified race walking style is more efficient and more enjoyable for most people. It will require about a month to adapt to the new style. The entire body should be loose and flexible at all times while walking to achieve the utmost efficiency. Walking then becomes sheer joy. Begin by taking a shorter stride than usual, landing on the heel with the toes up in the air (no high heels!) and loosely locking the knee. Keep all movements free and easy. As walking is as natural as eating and sleeping, the rest of your body will automatically follow your stride, with the upper body in reverse from the lower parts (when the left foot is forward, the right arm will be forward and vice versa). When you master the modified race walking style and you wish to go faster, your step will automatically lengthen. Just put the forward heel down easily, without effort, with the knee locked, and all else will follow. As your stride becomes faster your hands and forearms will tend to come up higher. In race walking circles it is said to be better to not cross the hands beyond the midline. Teaching this modified race walking style to all who are interested is my personal contribution to the walking art.

Walking offers many things—adventure, companionship, solitude; a time to think, a time to listen, relaxation, an enhanced appreciation of nature's wonders, improved mental and physical health, increased chances to achieve longevity, appetite control and weight control. Many of the great philosophers, statesmen, thinkers, writers, artists and world leaders have been dedicated walkers and have found inspiration in their daily walks. Perhaps meetings of world leaders would be more productive if walking in the fresh air in pleasant surroundings were included in their schedule of conferences instead of sitting and deliberating in stuffy, smoke-filled rooms.

You know they say, "The best things in life are free," and walking is a free gift. I recommend it to you and wish you many years of carefree walking.

The author, Dr. Charles Serritella, is a dedicated walker and his race walking competition events have found him logging thousands of miles over the past 50 years. Doc was a personal friend of Bernarr Macfadden, the famous publisher and "the father of physical culture" in the United States. The Macfadden Health Walks were held each year from 1935 through 1943. Here's how Serritella recalls the various events—

"Most of the hikes were of two weeks' duration and covered distances ranging from 298 to 410 miles. The 1939 walk took four weeks and totalled 640 miles, from Philadelphia to Dansville, N.Y., where we took a three-day rest at the unique Physical Culture Hotel, then on to the World's Fair in Flushing, N.Y.

"I was the trainer for the hikes and took care of the blisters, sore feet, and aching muscles. It is noteworthy that no one ever complained of a headache on health walks.

"It was also my privilege to have been a friend of one of the world's greatest long-distance walkers—James Hocking. Jim used to join us on our trail hikes in northern New Jersey in the forties. At that time, Jim was in his eighties.

"Jim broke many world records. When he was 68, he established a walking record of 17 days from New York to Chicago, a distance of 1,025 miles, breaking the record of another world-famous walker, E. P. Weston, by one day.

"He walked the Appalachian Trail and across the United States four or five times. He lived to a ripe old age of 101."

20

THE SECRET TO HEALTHY FEET

by Dr. Frank J. Garofalo

It is indeed ironical that the American people, being perhaps the most highly educated and informed on the face of the earth are also the most confused and indecisive in regard to good health. Although all of us have an idea of what good health is or should be, to each of us it means something different, depending on our age, physical activities, and present and past health status. For example, good health to a long-distance runner would mean the ability to run long races without fatigue, yet good health to a person in his late seventies would mean being able to do his daily chores, drive the car or have the vision to read a book. So, what is this elusive thing called good health that everyone knows about and yet finds hard to define?

Regardless of our definition of good health, I'm sure we would all include the following:

1. Freedom from pain
2. Unrestricted physical activity
3. Freedom from anxiety
4. A feeling of well-being

Now that we have some common definition of good

health, what can we do to keep our feet healthy?

Do you know the average adult will walk over a thousand miles a year? Multiply that by the life span and you will have walked around the world quite a few times. If we treat our feet well, we can expect to walk this distance in fine style.

The epitome of medical advancement is the prevention of disease. If we know the cause, we can then avoid illness. Today we know that many foot disorders can be prevented or minimized by early diagnosis and prompt, accurate treatment.

Flat foot deformity. Of all the deformities seen in the foot, none is as neglected and misdiagnosed as "flat feet." A child with a flat foot has a congenital-familial deformity which, if not diagnosed and treated early, will lead to secondary deformities. This can lead to a lifetime of pain and disability. Quite often the child with flat feet goes unnoticed by the parents and, surprisingly, sometimes by his own doctor because the child has no pain. Sometimes parents will bring their child to be examined because "his feet look funny," or "his ankles roll in."

The children with flat feet who are left untreated grow into their early teens with arch pain, painful heels and knees—experienced when they participate in sports. Later on in their middle years they suffer the secondary disabling deformities of bunions, contracted toes (hammer toes), painful corns and callouses on the balls of the feet and develop heel spurs. Disability by this time has become a major factor and surgery may be necessary to alleviate pain and to correct the situation.

Occasionally, with no medical treatment, the bunion deformity becomes severe and the big toe joint begins to wear out resulting in a stiff and painful arthritic joint. This will cause the patient to limp and it becomes impossible for him to bend his foot. To reduce the amount of pain and disability, part or all of the large toe joint must be surgically excised and a silicone prosthetic (artificial joint) implanted. So one can see that the usually overlooked flat foot can have grave consequences if neglected.

Treatment of flat foot consists of stabilizing the arch of the foot. This is accomplished by controlling excess motion in the joints comprising the arch as well as the abnormal motion of the bones just below the ankle. Special plastic arch supports called "orthotics" are commonly used to support the foot and allow the bones to grow normally.

Overlapping toes. Another congenital deformity is overlapping of the toes. When infants are found to have this condition, it can be easily corrected by very gently straightening the overlapping (or underlapping) toe and taping it to the adjacent toe. The normal toe thus acts as a splint and helps in realigning the deformed toe. The tape should be changed daily and great care must be taken that the tape is not too tight so as to impede circulation. Uncorrected over- or underlapping toes frequently form painful corns due to pressure.

Ingrowing nails. There are many causes of ingrowing nails.

1. Improperly cutting the nail too short or leaving a jagged piece of nail beneath the skin.

2. Tight, short or frayed shoes which press the flesh surrounding the nail against the borders of the nail.

3. Large shoes. If the shoes are too large the foot will slip forward in the shoe, causing the end of the nail to dig into the tip of the toe.

4. Elastic stockings which compress the toes, pressing the skin against the nail borders.

There is only one way to correctly trim a toenail and that is straight across. It's best not to cut the nail shorter than the end of the toe. As a final touch, smooth any rough edges.

Any suspected ingrown nail should be cleansed with

soap and water. Do not use hot water, for this will cause greater swelling and pain. Always seek professional care. Many a toe, leg and life have been lost because innocent-looking ingrown nails were treated by do-it-yourself amateur surgeons. Wear comfortable shoes that are neither too tight nor too loose. Check the inside of all your shoes by putting your hand inside to see if the lining of the shoe is bunched or frayed. If so, discard those shoes. A new pair of shoes is much less expensive than one or more visits to your doctor.

Congenital broad toes or congenital curved nails. Occasionally a child is born with very wide toes. This child's foot will develop ingrown nails because the average shoe is too narrow at the toe and thus the toes will be compressed in the shoe, causing the borders of the nail to cut into the skin adjacent to the nail. Congenital curved nails, also called "horse shoe" shaped nails, are so curved as to be bent upon themselves. These nails are raised and subject to shoe pressure from the top of the shoe.

Mycotic infections. These are also known as fungus infections and cause thickening and white discoloration of the nail. Irritation and pressure from the shoe or injury can start an acute infection which appears like an ingrown nail.

Athlete's foot infection. Athlete's foot is a superficial infection involving the skin of the foot. It usually occurs between the smaller toes at the webbing and the sole and inner arch areas of the foot. The infection causes burning, itching, fissuring and peeling of the skin. Frequently small blisters (vesicles) filled with a clear fluid will be present. Athlete's foot is caused by several varieties of fungi, which do not all respond to the same medication. This is the reason over-the-counter preparations do not always clear up the infection. Any infection, no matter how superficial, should be treated seriously, for a fungus infection can very rapidly turn into an acute bacterial infection.

Treatment of athlete's foot should begin by cleansing the infected area with mild soap and warm (not hot) water. Dry gently with a clean towel which must not be used for other parts of the body—otherwise you will spread the fungus. The foot should be aired so it will heal. Avoid wearing tennis shoes, plastic or suede shoes, boots and Hush-Puppy-type shoes. Rubber thongs and stretch socks will also aggravate the infection by allowing the perspiration and moisture to build up and spread the infection to surrounding areas. Seek professional help as soon as possible.

Soggy Feet. This condition is prevalent with teenagers. The skin at the ends of the toes peel and the calloused heels and soles become pitted. Parents complain that the children's feet smell. The skin is blanched and moist due to long, humid hours in athletic shoes. Despite the protestations by the parents as to their present state of social and hygienic unacceptability, the children's feet actually do not hurt.

This minor skin condition is caused by excessive movement in the shoe during rigorous physical activity and from the ensuing excessive perspiration. Chemical irritation from the shoes softens the skin, making it more subject to rubbing. Athletic shoes are largely made up of synthetic materials. The perspiration leeches out organic acids from these materials which can irritate the moist skin as well as alter the acidity of the skin. Soggy feet can lead to dermatitis and to athlete's foot infection.

To prevent soggy feet, avoid wearing athletic shoes for prolonged periods. Change shoes and socks after sports activities and allow the feet to air out. To reduce moisture, dust the inside of shoes with foot powder before wearing. Try alternating shoes that you wear so they can air out before you wear them again.

Planter warts. This is a benign, often painful, skin lesion that is caused by a minute virus. This virus is usually innoculated into the skin by way of a small cut or abrasion. Since viruses thrive in moist areas, most people contract the virus at the beach or swimming pools. Warts consist of small nerve endings and blood vessels which proliferate and become rounded and lie superficially. Warts can be solitary or satellite lesions and grow from a single lesion. Multiple warts are called mosaic warts.

How can you get rid of warts? Well, they can be extremely resistant to treatment. There are many ways to treat warts but generally stubborn or recurrent warts require a surgical incision combined with chemical application. One ancient remedy calls for lemon in any amount diluted into your footbath water. I strongly disapprove of electro-cautery (electric needle) for treatment of warts because scar formations and painful permanent adhesions can occur.

To prevent warts, air your shoes. Dry your feet after coming from the pool or beach. Good nutrition is a preventive. Eat foods high in vitamins A, E, C and B-complex. These vitamins will help to build the natural resistance to infection.

Soft corns. One of the most painful conditions commonly found on the foot is the presence of soft corns between the smaller toes, especially between the fourth and fifth (baby) toes. Corns are thick, calloused lesions over a small, bony prominence. The bony prominence is either an enlarged joint or bone spur at the end of the toe. Corns are a result of chronic irritation from shoes that are too narrow or do not conform to shape and length of the smaller toes. High-heeled dress shoes can cause soft corns because the body weight is concentrated on the ball and lesser toes. Bunions and flat feet can also cause soft corns by compressing the toes together.

Professional care is important. Treatment begins with paring the corn and treating any infection. Do not use chemical preparations that you buy at the drug store. These products are highly caustic and can rapidly ulcerate the underlying normal skin—opening the area to massive infection. If the soft corn recurs, despite a change of shoes, see your professional.

Here's how to prevent soft corns. Make sure your shoes fit comfortably the instant you try them on. Do not expect to "break the shoes in." Poor-fitting shoes can cause irreversible damage to your feet.

Prevention is the keyword in good foot health. Take heed to good nutrition, sensible, correct-fitting shoes and becoming acquainted with your podiatrist for routine checkups. You can't afford to take your feet for granted. Your feet must last you a lifetime. Remember, there aren't any spares around.

ABOUT THE AUTHORS

Dr. Vernon J. Bittner is internationally recognized as a leader in Clinical Pastoral Education. He earned his doctorate in psychology and religion. He is currently director of the Department of Religion and Health at North Memorial Hospital in Minneapolis, Minnesota. His recent books are *Make Your Illness Count* and *You Can Help with Your Healing*, Augsburg Publishers.

Willa Vae Bowles, in addition to her writing commitments, conducts seminars in nutrition throughout the United States. She is the founder and director of Temple Treasures Ministries; she makes her home in Tulsa, Oklahoma.

Audrey Carli is a prolific writer of articles about health/fitness and has made a lifelong study of health maintenance. She resides in Stambaugh, Michigan.

Dr. John R. Cheydleur is a regular contributor to *Total Health* magazine. He is president of California Christian Institute, the Christian Behavioral Science Graduate School, Anaheim, California. He has received the Distinguished Service Award from both Kiwanis

International and the National Association of Social Workers.

Dr. Arnold Fox practices internal medicine and cardiology in Beverly Hills, and is the director of the American Institute of Health in Beverly Hills, California. He is also an assistant professor of medicine at the University of California, Irvine, California. He authored the "Beverly Hills Medical Diet."

Barry Fox is a writer and playwright who co-authors "The Dr.'s Report" for *Total Health* magazine.

Dr. Frank J. Garofalo is a podiatrist-surgeon in Canoga Park, California. He is a member of California and American Podiatry Associations, Diplomate of the American Board of Podiatric Surgery, and Fellow of the American College of Foot Surgeons (board eligible).

Dr. Eppie Hartsuiker is a registered dietician with the American Dietetic Association and lecturer-host on the "More Abundant Health" radio program. She received her doctorate (Dr. H., SC.) from Loma Linda University.

Dr. Susan Smith Jones is currently a fitness and health instructor at UCLA. She is on the advisory board for the International Academy of Holistic Health and Medicine (IAHHM) and the National Joggers Association (NJA). A widely published free-lance writer of health articles, Dr. Jones has appeared on the cover of national magazines as the example of her healthy philosophy, which she discloses in her book, *The Main Ingredients: Positive Thinking, Exercise and Diet*. She has a Ph.D. in nutrition and exercise.

Daniel Kubelka is a former football player and physical fitness instructor. Dan teaches physical education in the Los Angeles public school system.

Dr. Charles Serritella is close to retirement age—but he is still walking for health. His race-walking competition events have found him logging thousands of miles over the past 50 years. He is a recent winner, in his age class, at the Main Masters Championship 3,000-meter walk. He has an active chiropractic practice in Caribou, Maine.

Robin Tracy is a free-lance writer and journalist whose articles appear regularly in various periodicals. She has made a lifelong study of the sleep habits in humans and is currently a research executive at the Better Sleep Council of America.

Marion Wells is a writer of numerous syndicated articles and research director of the American Physical Fitness Research Institute, Los Angeles.

SUBSCRIBE TO

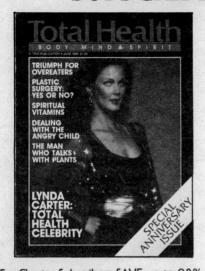

the most unique
holistic health
magazine